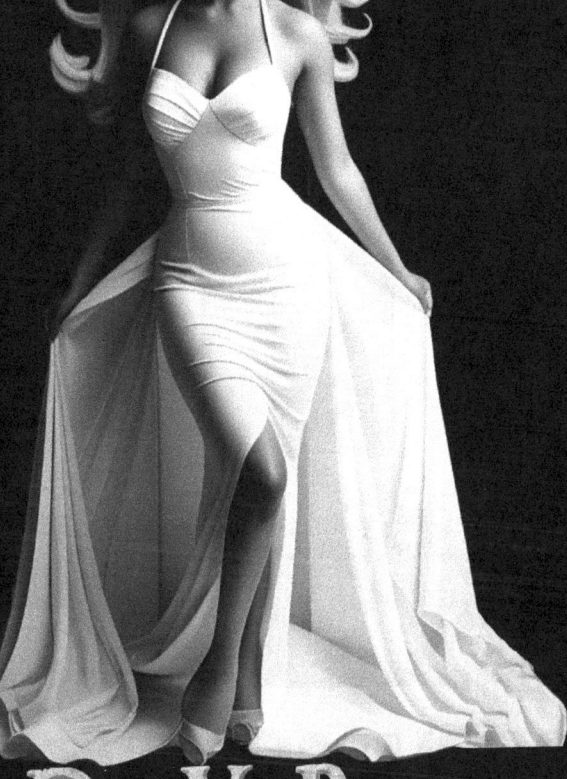

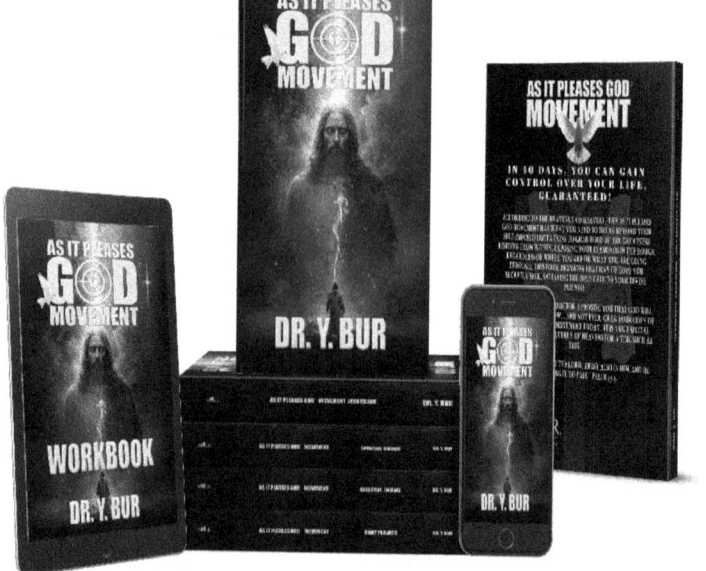

The *Bootylicious* Body
As It Pleases God®

The Secrets to Perfecting the Body of a Queen!

Copyright © 2025 by Dr. Y. Bur. All rights reserved.

Visit www.RoarPublishingGroup.com for more information. No part of this publication may be reproduced, stored in a retrieval system, or transmitted in any way by any means, electronic, mechanical, photocopy, recording, or otherwise, without the prior permission of the author, except as provided by USA copyright law.

Book design copyright © 2025 by R.O.A.R. International Group. All rights reserved.

R.O.A.R. Publishing Group
581 N. Park Ave. Ste. #725
Apopka, FL 32704
www.RoarPublishingGroup.com

Published in the United States of America
ISBN: 979-8-9990619-3-5
$22.88

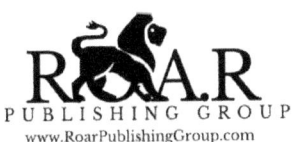

Send *As It Pleases God* ®
Book Series and Workbook Testimonies, Donations, Questions, or Orders to:

Dr. Y. Bur
R.O.A.R. Publishing Group
581 N. Park Ave. Ste. #725
Apopka, FL 32704
ROAR-58-2316
762-758-2316
Dr.YBur@gmail.com

Visit Us At:
AsItPleasesGodMovement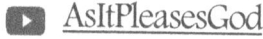
AsItPleasesGod

DrYBur.com
AsItPleasesGod.com

Please Donate

Please DONATE to this *Missionable Movement of God* as a GIVE-BACK to the Kingdom. Thanks for your support. Many Blessings.

AIPG Donation Link

Scan to Pay

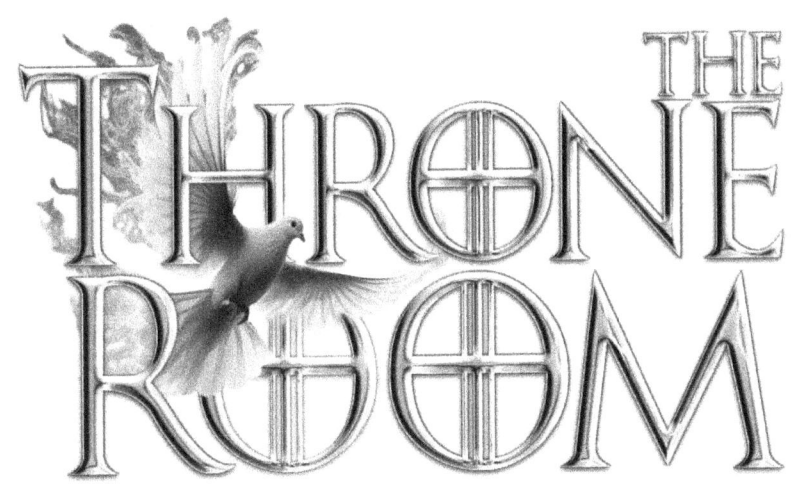

AS IT PLEASES GOD

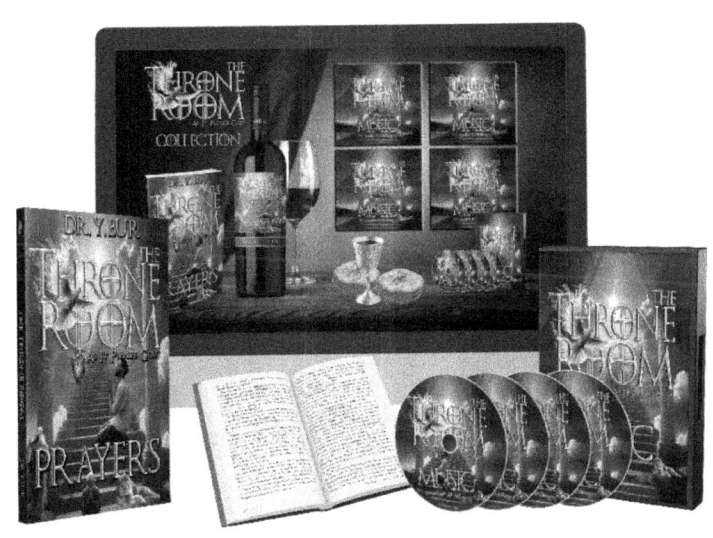

ASITPLEASESGOD.COM

Available Titles

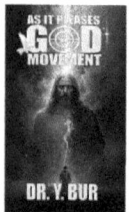 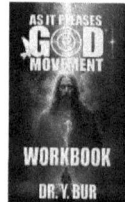 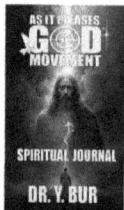 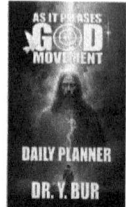 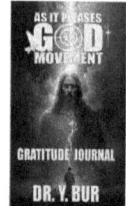

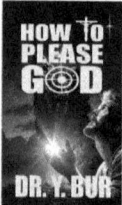 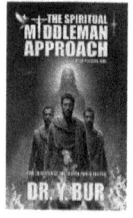 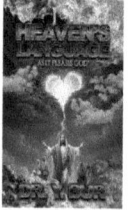 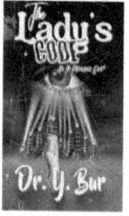 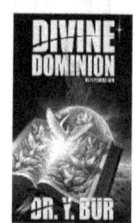

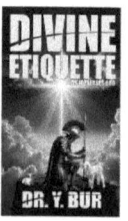 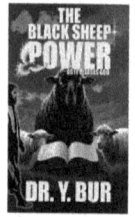 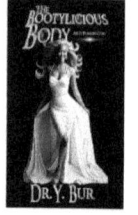 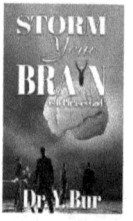 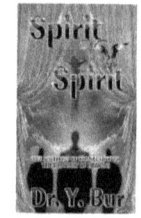

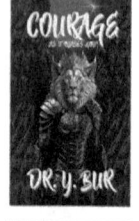 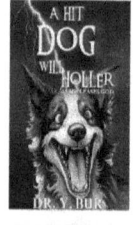 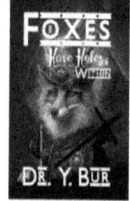 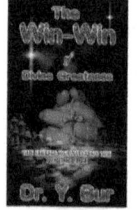 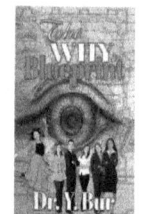

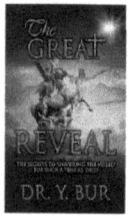 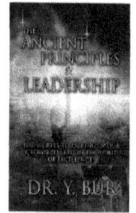 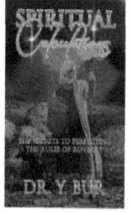 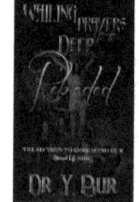 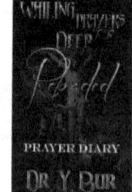

ASITPLEASESGOD.COM

Table of *Bootyliciousness*

INTRODUCTION 11
CHAPTER 1 19
   THE BOOTYLICIOUS PURPOSE 19
      Did God Make A Mistake? 24
      The Ultimate Goal 25
CHAPTER 2 27
   THE BOOTYLICIOUS SYSTEM 27
      Hormonal Imbalances 31
      A Queen's Branding 37
CHAPTER 3 45
   THE DIETAL SYSTEM 45
      The Approach 49
      Strike A Balance 51
      Hydration Matters 54
      Make Fitness Fun 58
      Diet and Exercise Wisdom 62
CHAPTER 4 63
   THE TEMPLE OF GOD 63
      The Power of Agreement 68
      Temple Maintenance 69
CHAPTER 5 83
   SELF-ACCEPTANCE 83

    Understanding Deception *85*
    Moving Forward *87*
    The Opportunity *92*
    In Purpose on Purpose *98*

CHAPTER 6 .... **103**
  Shadows of Greatness 103
    The Bullying of Children *105*
    Emotional Scars of a Child *110*
    No Bounds *113*

CHAPTER 7 .... **117**
  The Commitment 117
    Overcoming Vanity *121*
    Understanding Nutrition *127*
    The Body Speaks in Quinternity *135*

CHAPTER 8 .... **143**
  The Bootylicious Secrets 143
    The Natural Way *145*
    The Complainers *149*
    Can You Digest It? *151*
    The Queen's Secrets and Tips *153*

CHAPTER 9 .... **163**
  The Divine Canvas 163
    Harness Your Power *165*
    Avoid Judging *168*

CHAPTER 10 .... **171**
  The Bootylicious Freedom 171

The Fasting Process *176*
When to Start a Fast? *180*
Choices of Fasting *182*
The Chamber of Fasting *184*

CHAPTER 11 189

THE BOOTYLICIOUS MEAL PLAN 189
Smoothie Sensation 204
Jazz It Up 208

CHAPTER 12 211

NATURALLY BOOTYLICIOUS 211
The Bootylicious Connection 214

The Bootylicious Body Products

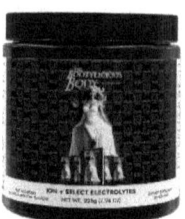
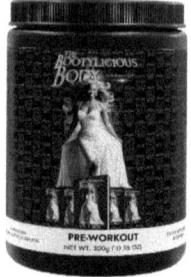
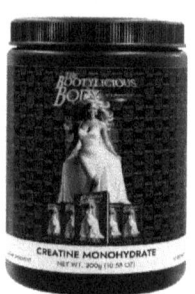
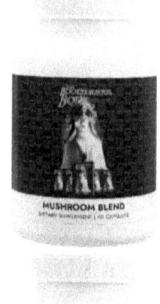
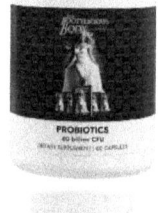
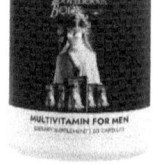
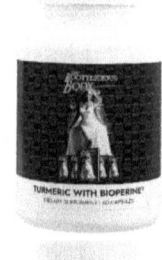
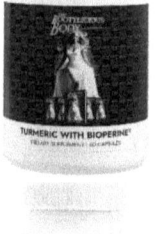
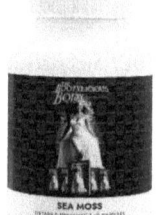
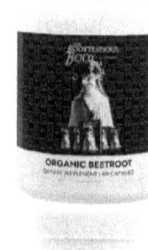
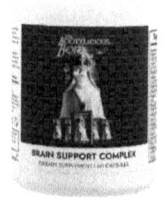
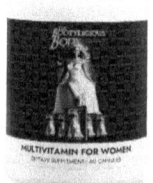
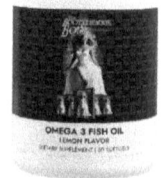
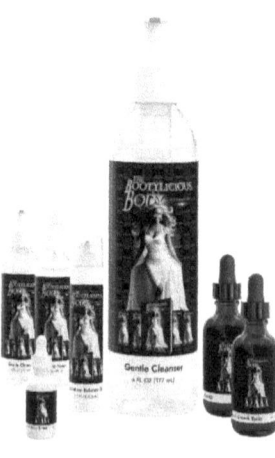
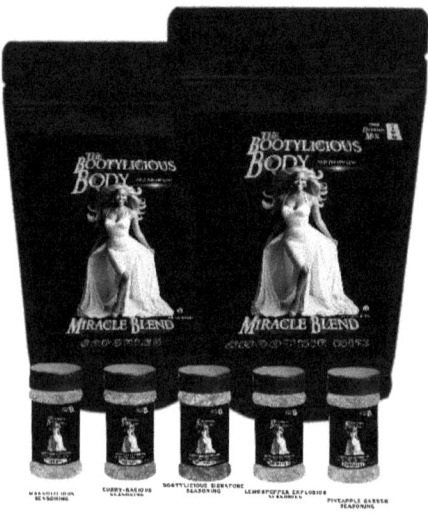

www.BootyliciousBody.com

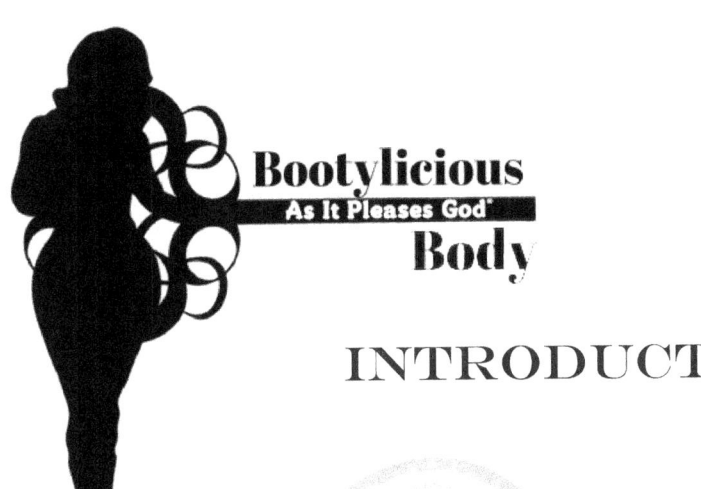

Bootylicious
As It Pleases God®
Body

INTRODUCTION

If you are looking to become someone else other than who you are, then this book is NOT for you. However, if you are looking to become the best version of yourself or to evolve into that true *Bootylicious Queen* from within, then keep reading. According to the Heavenly of Heavens, your joy and happiness will unveil itself when you love who you are at any weight, any size, any frame, any mindset, any culture, or any experience. In this book, *The Bootylicious Body: As It Pleases God®*, I will share with you how to develop this Profound Mindset to work with what you already have.

For the record, and before we go any further, God does not make mistakes, especially when He created you and the inner workings of your Divine Assets. Whether you like yourself or not, you must decide if you will become an asset or a liability in this world and beyond. Even if you do not understand this Spiritual Concept right now, know this: Inner Love is the foundation of the true *Bootylicious Queen* of yesterday, today, and forever more.

The *Bootylicious Queens* have been around since the beginning of time, even if we as a society fail to recognize their

Introduction

presence. In the Spirit of Excellence, a real, authentic *Bootylicious Queen* is not often recognized in today's society as being the woman of choice or chance. Instead, she tends to become recognized in the *Shadows of Greatness* by those who do not identify the value that she truly possesses from within. Yet, when she shines, her thickness becomes measured against her intelligence, which often causes her to be placed on the back burner or to become the last choice or the default mechanism.

What an insult to the dominant race of *Bootylicious Queens* that lurk in the shadows without owning their true curves. Society is painting an image of getting our curviness sucked out or tucked in to feed our sense of vanity. But, God forbid...the beauty of a *Bootylicious Queen* resides in her natural health, Spiritual Wellness, character traits, wise mindset, and healthy eating habits.

As 'Bootylicious Queens,' we are faced with many different issues in life, from the home front with family and relational or communicational qualms that are often left unresolved or hidden under something else. Then, as if this is not enough, we must deal with the forefront of what lies ahead while tackling the back alley of our traumatic pasts. In addition, we are still confronting the commitment factors to continue to move forward with little or no support or recognition while dealing with hurt, betrayal, abuse, confusion, and discrimination. All of which can take a toll on the human psyche, but all are doable in Christ Jesus. However, we, as women in the Eye of God, must know what to do, when to do it, how to do so, and why we are doing what we do.

For the record, this book is NOT about us spreading our cheeks to the highest bidder. It is designed to bring forth the True Queen from within while learning how to value the nookie without allowing everyone or anything into the cookie jar. When we consciously or unconsciously diminish our

Introduction

value, it will silently take a toll on our self-image and self-esteem by default, turning a True Queen into an insecure pauper of discontentment. For this reason, in the Eye of God, we will become a bottomless pit, lacking humility in a pool of jealousy, envy, pride, coveting, competitiveness, and comparison.

Self-image and self-esteem are major factors in how we deal with, overcome, and rebound when life is lifing. For many, losing weight is often easier said than done, especially when dealing with health challenges, bodily risks, and hormonal imbalances. Now, what I have found is that those who refuse to deal with their self-esteem or self-image issues tend to allow life just to happen without self-correcting or correcting the correctable.

For the above reasons, in this book, we deal with the Mind, Body, Soul, and Spirit to create a balance between these four components of Divine Stability. If we do not deal with them, *As It Pleases God*, one can have a banging body without emotional intelligence, or one can have emotional intelligence and cannot push the plate away. Then again, one can fear eating altogether to avoid gaining weight, not realizing we must eat to live. In addition, most of us do not know that the body will begin to eat itself in order to function, doing what it is designed to do. Still, we must do our part in this equation without developing a deaf ear to our reality. All of this is real, and it is happening before our very eyes.

Nevertheless, God wants us to become good stewards of every aspect of our being, including the release of good and bad hormones. But do not worry; this book is designed to break this information down into palatable, bite-sized information while taking a deeper look into our dietary challenges from a Divine Perspective.

Introduction

In a world where health trends shift as quickly as the seasons, it is not what we are eating that is causing our problems; it is more about what is eating us. Regardless of whether we are participating in diets high in protein, low in carbs, low in sugar, low in fat, veganism, or anything in between, we are all different. Thus, we will all have varying emotional and psychological relationships with people, places, things, and, most of all, food.

According to our Divine Design, we will not all like the same things based on our senses, taste buds, experiences, cultural backgrounds, coping mechanisms, and triggers. In my opinion, this is similar to everyone having a different fingerprint, eyeprint, footprint, mindprint, and Spiritual Blueprint. We must know the difference, *As It Pleases God*, to ensure we are dealing with our correct bodily setpoint, especially when dealing with stress, anxiety, loneliness, or depression.

What if we are not stressed, anxious, lonely, or depressed? When living life, we will experience them all—no one is exempt. We must know how to deal with them according to our DNA, or they can manifest in unhealthy eating habits, pretenses, or negative bodily responses, leading to obesity, eating disorders, and gastrointestinal problems. To be clear, this is nothing to be ashamed of—the time is now to address these issues without looking down on ourselves or others for their status or condition.

In this book, I am speaking from experience. I am not finger-pointing or discrediting anyone for the choices they are making; I am extending Divine Wisdom from the Heavens Above. What I had to endure to get this information is not something I would wish upon my worst enemy. With the correct heart and mind posture from the Heavenly of Heavens, I give unto thee. As I embark on this Spiritual Journey of sharing my personal stories and insights, after being called all

Introduction

types of names, I make it a priority to come from a place of integrity, clarity, and understanding.

One thing is for sure: Life is a tapestry of experiences, stories, and revelations, woven with threads of duality, both good and bad, right and wrong, just and unjust, joy and sorrow, belief and unbelief, or wins and losses. All of which provide us an opportunity to choose, reflect, and grow with free will. This beacon of light symbolically provides us with a navigating Spiritual Compass of our shadows to seek clarity, understanding, regrafting, and elevation amidst whatever with whomever.

As you dive into the pages of this book, I encourage you to approach it with an open mind and heart through the echoes of your past, present, and future. Why is this so important? Life has a way of speaking, and you only need to listen as it guides you toward your own revelations. Here is what you can glean from this book, but not limited to such:

- ☐ Unveil or extract your Divine Purpose.
- ☐ Establish the how-to in building a System.
- ☐ Develop a Spiritual Mindset, *As It Pleases God*.
- ☐ How to better understand your WHY in life.
- ☐ Create a pleasing lifestyle of authenticity.
- ☐ How to eat properly.
- ☐ How to create meal plans.
- ☐ The power of cleansing your body.
- ☐ The secrets of Kingdom Etiquette.
- ☐ The best ways to get your body moving.
- ☐ Learn the secrets to becoming really confident.
- ☐ Understand the power of owning your truth.
- ☐ How to overcome the lies you tell yourself.
- ☐ How to deal with your psyche, *As It Pleases God*.

Introduction

- ☐ How to master or maximize the power hidden in the Mind, Body, Soul, and Spirit Quaternity.
- ☐ The secrets to gaining Divine Wisdom.
- ☐ How to bring forth the Virtuous Woman from within.
- ☐ How to maximize the Quinternity Effect of personal development from the Heavenly of Heavens.

In the Eye of God, the *Queens of Bootyliciousness* are powerful, influential women, and you too, have that Divine Birthright! When you cultivate the willpower to overcome excuses, you are then able to rebound from people, places, and things that may have gotten you temporarily off track on how to eat clean and the importance of moving your body. For the most part, if this book has found you, you are indeed a *Bootylicious Queen*, and it is my reasonable service to educate you on your NATURAL roots to ensure that you are able to live the healthy lifestyle of your Queenship.

The question is, 'Can we be sexy and on fire for God simultaneously?' Yes, we can. In the Kingdom of God, we do not have to walk around looking beat down or unkempt unless we desire to do so. My whole life, I have been ostracized, abused, rejected, body-shamed, and called all types of names for being cute, curvy, thick, and sexy. Walking around with a whole lot of junk in my trunk (having a big butt) does not justify being mistreated, especially by those who claim to be Believers. God created me as a Curvy Girl for a reason, and I was not going to allow anyone to make me ungodly or shatter my confidence to satiate their insecurities or internal qualms.

In taking this learning experience a step further, I stood back and watched some of the charactorial assassination culprits swing it high and low, doing things behind closed doors that would get a serious side-eye from God. Even I had

Introduction

enough sense to know that looking like something or someone with zero action or execution and doing (such as taking action) are two different things. In my opinion, this is similar to labeling someone guilty without any action occurring by someone who is fully engaged in what they are blaming others for doing, without a justifiable cause. Nevertheless, beyond a shadow of a doubt, while they were playing dirty, I knew how to keep my legs closed without getting into the mud or outing their dirty laundry. To say the least, I was kind to others while they behaved as if they had zero home training.

Above all, although I was not perfect, I was repenting, respectful, forgiving, and merciful, even when they wronged me in a bad way, as they walked around without a conscience. For me, I did not understand how they confused being sexy with being ungodly, especially when they were behaving like hellions on wheels, exhibiting zero Fruits of the Spirit. Their unrealistic view of HOLINESS and BEAUTY could have caused me to doubt myself. But instead, it inspired me to cultivate a mindset of positivity that extends beyond appearances and opinions.

More importantly, I hold no grudges against them...for it is through their short-sightedness that enabled me to become the woman that I am today. All in all, God allowed them to sharpen my Spiritual Skills and Ingenuity, enabling me to glean the Timely Information and Divine Wisdom needed to become Purposefully Effective and Kingdomly Usable, confounding human understanding.

The Bootylicious Body: As It Pleases God® serves as a guide, illuminating your path through prayer, meditation, repentance, character development, conscious living, and effectively using the Fruits of the Spirit. As we rise above the noise and distractions of life, this book is not only a Divine Testament to my Spiritual Journey but also a TRIBUTE to all

Introduction

those who seek to learn, grow, thrive, and sow back into the Kingdom when called upon.

In this ultimate guide to embracing your *Bootylicious* self, I extend my hand to you on this Divine Journey in the Spirit of TOGETHERNESS. Embracing your unique shape can be liberating, empowering, and a powerful statement of self-love and self-acceptance, regardless of what others think or feel about you. With a *Bootylicious Mindset* of Gracefulness, let us explore the depths of your heart and soar toward the Divine Truths that await, *Spirit to Spirit.*

According to the Heavenly of Heavens, your body is a *Divine Canvas* of strength, resilience, fortitude, and beauty, especially when it embodies the *Bootylicious Spirit* of loving the skin you are in. And, regardless of where you are in life, your condition, your status, or the challenges you are faced with, you are a Divine Masterpiece, and by no means should you ever give up on yourself. Remember, you are a work-in-progress, so if you fall short one day, get back on track the next day.

As a Word to the Wise, in the Kingdom, faith, love, hope, obedience, humility, confidence, and courage are the most attractive qualities in the Eye of God. So, stand tall, loving every inch of your *Bootylicious* Mind, Body, Soul, and Spirit, and watch how God will transform your life with this one book. Guaranteed. You deserve it!

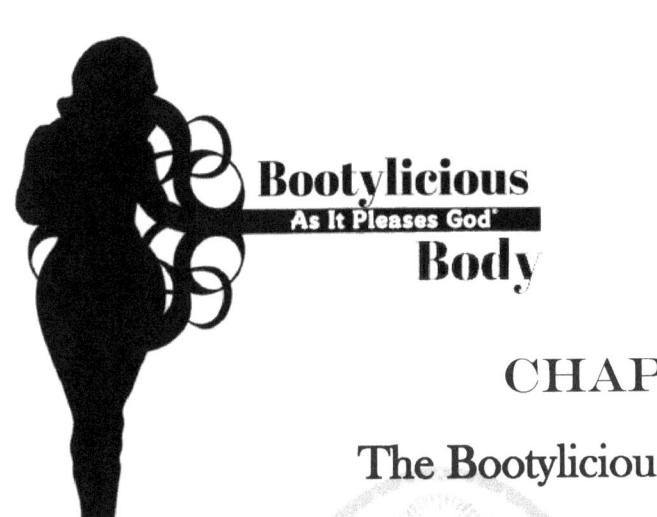

Bootylicious Body
As It Pleases God®

CHAPTER 1
The Bootylicious Purpose

In recent years, a cultural shift has given rise to a wave of Divine Movements aimed at celebrating self-love, body positivity, purposefulness, and reclaiming our virtuousness. As Women of Stature, in the celebration of our curves and femininity, *The Bootylicious Body: As It Pleases God* challenges societal norms that often dictate biased beauty standards, giving birth to *The Bootylicious Purpose*. With the blending of Spiritual Empowerment and Divine Purpose, along with the celebration of our Temples, *As It Pleases God*, it definitely changes the rules of the game on any level or playing field. All of which gives us an opportunity to bring forth the Greatness that is already trapped within our loins.

The core message of *The Bootylicious Purpose* is simple yet profound: Love yourself while loving your curves and all... while healthily defining beauty on your own terms. In the Eye of God, every woman, good, bad, or indifferent, is worthy of love and acceptance—just as she is without being shamed, humiliated, rejected, ostracized, or excluded for not meeting societal standards. By reshaping our perceptions and mindsets from pleasing men to *As It Pleases God*, help us in advocating for inclusion, diversity, and healthiness.

In this chapter, the goal is to gain the know-how to set powerful examples for future generations. So, let us begin with the WHY of *The Bootylicious Body: As It Pleases God*.

The Bootylicious Purpose initiates and promotes body positivity, creating a safe, supportive space for curvy women to connect, share their experiences, and uplift each other, *As It Pleases God*. Through our online forums, workshops, seminars, personal storytelling, and events, participants can discuss challenges they face, celebrate victories, and share tips on self-acceptance. This supportive network combats the culture of comparison and fosters genuine connections, reminding women that they are not alone in their journey.

The innate desire to inspire curvy women has somehow fallen to the ground as we focus on labeling them as obese, perpetuating unrealistic ideals, goals, and desires. Then again, as my ear has been to the ground, the gaslighting has gotten out of control, as we treat curvy women as if it is some sort of plague if she is a thick chick or as if God made a mistake.

In addition, mockery or insulting others has become commonplace under the guise of attempts to help while hurting those we claim to love, which can take a toll on their mental health. By offering resources on body positivity, self-love, and mental health support, the initiative addresses the emotional challenges that curvy women often face.

When we do not struggle with that same issue, it is easy to judge and point the finger without understanding the underlying factors associated with curvaceousness. How do I know? Experience is the best teacher...I have been on both sides of this issue to bring my findings back to the Kingdom of God about this matter, stifling the obesity narrative. While visual representation dominates our social feeds and media, it

The Bootylicious Purpose

is imperative to develop confidence in our curves and unapologetically love ourselves with a healthy mindset to make better decisions about our well-being.

In the narrow manmade standards of beauty, curvy women face unique challenges of multiple stereotypes belittling their worth. For this reason, in the *Bootylicious Body: As It Pleases God*, we must discuss how curvy women can navigate the unique challenges that come with falling outside of normal societal expectations.

In the Eye of God, beauty comes in all different shapes, sizes, purposes, and DNA structures, even if we do not understand His reasoning for their existence.

According to the Heavenly of Heavens, anything created with the Breath of Life, be it humans, animals, pathogens, or whatever, we are all grafted into a categorical seismic edifice, even if we disagree with God's rationale or reasoning for doing so. Are pathogens grafted into the Breath of Life? Absolutely. If pathogens can take human life, it means they possess more power than what meets the eye, right?

What do pathogens have to do with anything? In *The Bootylicious Purpose*, negativity becomes its own pathogen, causing and carrying disease among the brethren, weakening or infecting their immune systems. In order to defend ourselves from a cryptic takeover, we must interject positivity, continuous growth, nutritional understanding, and purposefulness. Keep in mind that in the Animal Kingdom, they do not have an issue with criticizing and degrading God's Divine Creation. Instead, they focus on establishing and preserving their Bloodlines, doing what they were called to do.

In or out of the Kingdom of God, there is no one-size-fits-all manual for anything when dealing with our Heaven on Earth Experiences. When we lack the motivation or the esteem needed to lose weight, transforming the Mind, Body,

The Bootylicious Purpose

Soul, and Spirit, we will find ourselves falling into a cryptic place of wallowing in hurts, atrocities, and betrayals of the past. Now, through the Hand of God or as fate would have it, this is where the treasure trove of Divine Wisdom and Insights in *The Bootylicious Body* comes into play, serving as a Guiding Light, *As It Pleases God*.

My *Bootylicious Queen*, the motivation and the answers that you are seeking are hidden in the pages of *The Bootylicious Body*. The information is not hidden on purpose...it is just that every *Bootylicious Queen* is different, with various wants, needs, traumas, and experiences, so the answers that you need may not be in one place.

On the other hand, when dealing with the intertwining of your Mental, Physical, Emotional, and Spiritual Landscapes, the information that you may have mastered could be the information needed for another *Bootylicious Queen*. In the Eye of God, it is crucial to delve deep into your past and confront the emotions tied to those experiences. If not, you will begin to ignore or overlook the triggers associated with negative emotions, desires, habits, thoughts, beliefs, and reactions, contributing to a negative self-image.

Listen, the true *Bootylicious Queens* have a pact to help each other based on the Law of Reciprocity, redefining narratives. We are all sisters in Christ Jesus, and we all have a platform to help others. We are all great in our own right, and the time has come for us to own our rightful place with our curves and all!

On this note, *The Bootylicious Body: As It Pleases God*® offers a pathway not just to weight loss, but to self-acceptance, self-elevation, and self-love extended outwardly with the Fruits of the Spirit. How do we make this make sense? When we use the Fruits of the Spirit...Love, Joy, Peace, Patience, Kindness, Goodness, Faithfulness, Gentleness, and Self-Control in our

The Bootylicious Purpose

Bootyliciousness, our character traits will begin to align us with Kingdom Principles, Standards, Poshness, and Etiquette by default to sustain our transformation.

Does the use of the Fruits of the Spirit really make a difference? Absolutely! In my opinion, it is very disheartening to have a banging body with bad character and rotten fruit all over the place. So, regardless of our body types or sizes, the goal in *The Bootylicious Body: As It Pleases God* is to possess good character traits and fruits while behaving Christlike.

According to the Heavenly of Heavens, each step you take is a Testament to your strength and resilience, or the lack thereof. Nevertheless, in this book, we are going to remain on the positive side of the spectrum, building ourselves from the inside out, *As It Pleases God*. In order to do so, we must add God into the equation of our *Bootyliciousness*. Of course, some naysayers would argue that we should not add God into the equation of our *Bootyliciousness*. They may also advise that we should keep God separate from our Spiritual Discourses regarding beauty, body image, allure, or attractiveness. But, as a *Bootylicious Queen* of the Most High God, I personally beg to differ, especially when He created us in His Divine Image.

If we read the Song of Solomon in the Bible, taking a deep dive into the rich, alluring text, we would sing a different tune regarding admirable expressions such as luscious fruits, flowing flowers, and striking landscapes. All of which are worthy of celebration and respect, with a paradigm shift. The Song of Solomon is a poetic narrative, painting vivid pictures of the physicalities of love for Him, ourselves, and others without becoming like a brood of vipers full of hypocrisy, internal corruption, debauchery, and moral failure.

What does the Song of Solomon have to do with the brood of vipers? As *Bootylicious Queens*, our inner thoughts, feelings, and words are connected to our *Bootyliciousness*, creating an antidote (The Healing), poison (The Toxicity or Plague), or venom (The Cycle of Death) of our choosing. Here is what Matthew 12:34 asks us: *"Brood of vipers! How can you, being evil, speak good things? For out of the abundance of the heart the mouth speaks."* Whereas, with the Song of Solomon, we can glean profound insights into the celebration of the human body, our desires, and idealistic love, turning our natural propensities into an alluring POWER from the Ancient of Days.

Did God Make A Mistake?

In a world fixated on physical appearances, the one thing we must understand is that God did not give women bigger bums for no reason. Then again, it is easy to forget that our bodies are gifts bestowed upon us for varying reasons. Now, if we do not know our reasons, it is time to get in the know, especially when becoming peaceful with ourselves and our reason for being with dignity and grace. With *The Bootylicious Body: As It Pleases God*, if we dare to align our character with Kingdom Standards, the Divine Illumination of a woman's poshness will come forth without us having to overdo it or expose ourselves.

The primitive question is, 'How do you know if you are a *Bootylicious Queen*?' The *Bootylicious Queens* are unique. They are very distinctive in nature, character, and appearance. She has a sense of style about her that causes others to want to emulate her. *Bootylicious Queens* are usually not small-framed women; they are typically very solid in weight. Their bodies are well-built, and they do not have a problem exuding power and authority. Nevertheless, society has a way of trying to brainwash the *Bootylicious Queens* into thinking that they are not good enough, thin enough, pretty enough, healthy enough, and the list goes on. But, my *Bootylicious Queen*, I am here to help you reclaim your crown.

The Bootylicious Purpose

Even if you have a few extra pounds on your body, it does not matter! A *Bootylicious Queen* has a certain type of dietal regimen that caters to the health of that particular body type. Although doctors tend to label a *Bootylicious Queen* as obese, which may not be the case at all. The ultimate goal is health. If you are eating clean food and moving your body with a great bill of health, then you have no need to worry.

As a *Bootylicious Queen*, your appearance is of great importance. If you are adorning your appearance for someone else, you are out of order, and the satisfaction will not last! People-pleasing will turn into self-hate if you are not careful about this sort of behavior. It is for this reason, we have those who are trying to lose more weight when they do not need to. Losing too much weight is not good for your health, and it is not attractive. With all due respect, if you are already thin and you still feel fat, you need to consult your doctor.

The Ultimate Goal

As a word of caution, any weight-related health problems or complications due to extreme dieting may be irreversible. Therefore, your goal should always be to remain healthy. There is no need to be ashamed of your body, dodging the mirror, or hiding from the people you love. You are the best you that you have. As a *Bootylicious Queen*, it is time to develop your own weight loss plan and fitness regimen, as well as a healthy plan of action to achieve your goals.

Here are a few questions used in developing a Bootylicious Body Mindset, *As It Pleases God*, but not limited to such:

- ☐ How do you feel about your body?
- ☐ What is your response when looking in the mirror?
- ☐ When do these feelings arise?

The Bootylicious Purpose

- ☐ Where do you experience these feelings?
- ☐ How do these feelings affect you?
- ☐ Why do you think you feel this way?
- ☐ What can you do to overcome these feelings?
- ☐ Are you grateful or appreciative of your body?
- ☐ Do you view your body as the Temple of God?
- ☐ Does your self-confidence increase or deflate when viewing your body?

What is the purpose of asking ourselves these questions? If we do not query ourselves, the psyche will tend to hide valuable information from us, causing us to self-sabotage or self-destruct when we least expect it. In addition, if we fail to query our actions, thoughts, beliefs, or desires, the lust of the eyes, the lust of the flesh, and the pride of life will operate at full throttle, making our *Bootyliciousness* a sour patch. Is this not a little insensitive? Maybe or maybe not, but what is more insensitive is to have all the external workings, and the moment we open our mouths, the show is over.

If we do not possess the wherewithal to keep or sustain what we attract, it is time to put in the work, doing a charactorial overhaul, *As It Pleases God*. Clearly, I am not pointing the finger here. I had to do a charactorial overhaul myself, so I do not settle for excuses when needing a checkup from the neck up. Instead, I provide a roadmap to help you to help yourself with documented facts, Divine Wisdom, and palatable understanding that really works when dealing with the Mind, Body, Soul, Spirit, and eating regimens. So, let us move on to *The Bootylicious System* to give you a better understanding of how to make your body a Kingdomly Certified Powerhouse, Brickhouse, or Temple of God, *As It Pleases Him*.

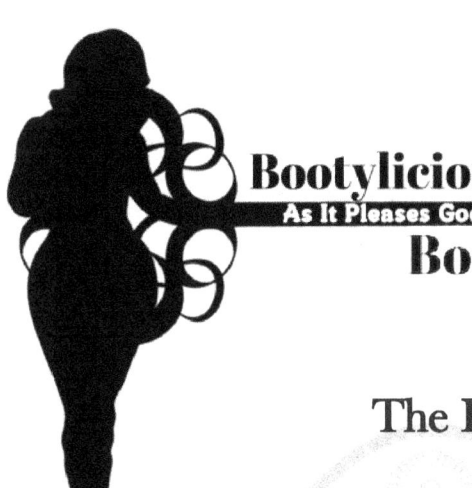

CHAPTER 2
The Bootylicious System

When it comes to the world of dieting, you will find that there are many diets, weight loss plans, fitness gurus, or bogus gimmicks on the market. However, one of the 'best kept' secrets until now is the Divine System hidden within *The Bootylicious Body: As It Pleases God*®.

What makes *The Bootylicious System* so different? Simply put, we add God into the equation Mentally, Physically, Emotionally, and Spiritually. In the Eye of God, it is not wise to fix the body while overlooking the Mind, ignoring our Emotions, and downplaying our Spirituality. In the Kingdom, it is a recipe for disaster because we are Spiritual Beings having a human experience.

According to the Heavenly of Heavens, by overlooking the Earthen Vessel that already lies within, we will function at a deficit or overcompensate in some areas of our lives, especially if we are out of purpose, disobedient, or negligent. How so? For example, suppose we are a little shaky mentally or emotionally, and we can control our weight. In this case, that is the area we will focus on the most, with imbalanced perspectives and biases, looking down on or mistreating those who obviously appear not to control their weight. Unfortunately, this is a silent way to make us feel better about ourselves when lacking mental or emotional intelligence, secretly or openly. If we do not call this out for what it is, we will continue to lie to ourselves about the rotten and mangled fruits we are leaving behind.

Then again, if we cannot control our weight but are well-to-do in our finances, we will place more attention on wealth building, dogging out those who appear to have less. Unfortunately, both analogies come with a double-edged sword, so it is only wise to avoid judging what we do not understand. In addition, we must avoid mistreating others who appear beneath us.

Why should we exercise caution when judging or calling people out, especially when having free will? First, we do not know another man's story. Secondly, negative or debauched seeds bear fruit in due season. Thirdly, if we do not have it all together, then what is the purpose of degrading God's precious sheep? Should we not be guiding them or sharing information that is uplifting, palatable, and helpful? Absolutely!

My *Bootylicious Queen*, we are a beacon of light to the world. If we are dimming the light of the next man without just cause or operating with half of the information without asking fact-finding questions, then we have work to do Mentally, Physically, Emotionally, and Spiritually. Why must we put in the work? In the Eye of God, we can have it all, primarily if we approach all things with a Divine System, *As It Pleases Him*, with an understanding.

In establishing and maintaining our Kingdom Status, *As It Pleases God*, it is imperative not to place image over possessing positive character traits. If we do, masks will form, invoking

The Bootylicious System

layers of pretense. Plus, this is not what this book is about...we are here to develop authenticity with a *Bootylicious System* that can withstand the tests of time.

As a *Bootylicious Queen*, you are an ICON in your own right. You are the warrior over your DESTINY. You are the warrior over your BODY. You are the warrior over your SOUL. You are the warrior over your MIND. And, most of all, you are the warrior over your SPIRIT. When you lose contact with the warrior from within, you leave an opening, a longing, or a void that you will tend to fill with other things that take you away from the *Bootylicious Queen* from Within.

What is the purpose of having *The Bootylicious System* in place? As Women of Stature, our warfare comes in the form of a battle with the bulge, a battle with our health, a battle with our minds, a battle with our emotions, a battle of our sexual natures, a soulish battle with our traumas, a battle in our homes, a battle with our children, and a Spiritual Battle to say the least. If one does not understand the fullness of their *Bootylicious Nature*, they will miss the mark when it comes down to understanding the true nature from within and the instinctual nature of what is taking place from within and around them.

In developing a *Bootylicious Mindset* with a foolproof system of conveyance, we must effectively query ourselves, *As It Pleases God*. Listed below are a few questions to get our inner voice to speak, developing our *Bootylicious Mindsets* to get an understanding of what is taking place within the psyche. Nevertheless, when answering these questions, make sure you are documenting your answers in your *Bootylicious Journal*.

- ☐ What does having a *Bootylicious Body Mindset* mean to you personally?

The Bootylicious System

- ☐ How can a positive body image impact your overall mental health?
- ☐ In what ways can you align your fitness goals with your Spiritual Values?
- ☐ What practices can help you cultivate self-love?
- ☐ How does societal pressure influence your perception of a Bootylicious Body?
- ☐ What role does gratitude play in developing a healthy body image and mindset?
- ☐ How can you incorporate prayer or meditation into your eating and fitness routines?
- ☐ What are some ways to celebrate your body's achievements, regardless of societal standards?
- ☐ How can a strong support system enhance your journey towards a *Bootylicious Body Mindset*?
- ☐ What challenges do you face in reconciling body goals with living in a way that pleases God?
- ☐ How can you shift your focus from appearance to overall health and well-being?
- ☐ What is the importance of nourishing your body with healthy foods in this mindset?
- ☐ How does exercise or movement contribute to your Mental, Physical, Emotional, and Spiritual Wellness?
- ☐ In what ways can you use setbacks as opportunities for growth?
- ☐ How can you stay motivated to maintain a positive mindset despite external pressures?
- ☐ What scriptures or Spiritual Texts inspire you in your pursuit of a healthy mindset?
- ☐ How can you practice patience and kindness towards yourself during your eating and fitness journey?
- ☐ What does it mean to you to honor your body as a temple while pursuing a Bootylicious Body?

The Bootylicious System

- How can you distinguish between healthy ambition and an unhealthy obsession?
- What steps will you take today to align your body goals with your values and beliefs?

Most often, doctors link health complications with obesity, which is partially true and multifaceted. On the other side of this truth, we have the types of foods being consumed with low nutritional quality. In addition, we have poor diets, hormonal imbalances, genetics, stress levels, lifestyles, and physiological impacts of day-to-day living.

With or without our permission, our DNA can indeed influence our metabolisms, fat storage, and how our bodies respond to different foods. What does this mean? Even without our conscious consent, our complex genetic makeup plays an instrumental role in shaping our metabolic tendencies. This complex relationship would also include how we convert food, process nutrients, store energy, and ultimately, how we burn calories.

As *Bootylicious Queens*, the power of our Genetic Blueprint contains a direct link to our hormones, balancing them or creating an imbalance. Therefore, to safeguard our lineage, *As It Pleases God*, we must get a better understanding of how all of this impacts our health.

Hormonal Imbalances

How do we make all of this DNA and hormonal stuff make sense? In all simplicity, with *The Bootylicious System*, hormones such as insulin, leptin, and ghrelin all interact in ways that can either promote weight gain or facilitate weight loss. So, when life is lifing, it can become challenging to drop weight, even if

The Bootylicious System

we are eating clean and exercising. How do I know? Once again, experience makes the best teacher teach effectively with first-hand information.

In addition, we also must deal with stress-triggered hormones, such as, but not limited to:

- ☐ Cortisol (The Stress Hormone): The adrenal glands release Cortisol in response to stress. Unbeknown to some, Cortisol helps regulate various functions, including the metabolism, regulation of blood pressure, fat storage, and immune response. In addition, it also influences the appetite and cravings for high-calorie, sugary, and fatty foods. More importantly, some are allergic or sensitive to the release of this hormone without knowing it. Therefore, if we experience skin reactions, gastrointestinal issues, mood changes, or extreme fatigue, we must check with our doctor about this to avoid the adverse effects associated.

- ☐ Adrenaline (Epinephrine): This hormone is also released by the adrenal glands during stressful situations, leading to increased heart rate, blood pressure, and energy production, helping the body prepare for a 'fight or flight response.

- ☐ Norepinephrine: This hormone complements adrenaline and plays a role in the body's response to stress. It affects our attention span, response times, quick actions, and mood regulations, aiding in the body's alertness during stressful situations.

- ☐ Corticotropin-Releasing Hormone (CRH): Produced in the hypothalamus, CRH stimulates the release of adrenocorticotropic hormone (ACTH) from the

The Bootylicious System

pituitary gland, which in turn stimulates the adrenal glands to produce cortisol.

- ☐ Adrenocorticotropic Hormone (ACTH): This hormone is produced by the pituitary gland and plays a role in the stress response by stimulating cortisol production in the adrenal glands.

- ☐ Vasopressin (Antidiuretic Hormone): Released during stress, vasopressin plays a role in regulating water balance in the body and can affect blood pressure.

Without a true understanding of a person's situation or circumstance, we are conditioned to negatively label or reject God's prize creation for the lack of understanding.

How do we counteract these stressful hormones? According to the Heavenly of Heavens, we must begin using the Fruits of the Spirit and behave Christlike, *As It Pleases God*. Once done, the body will naturally balance itself out by releasing happy hormones, such as Endorphins, Dopamine, Serotonin, and Oxytocin (The Love Hormone). These are neurotransmitters and hormones that contribute to feelings of happiness and well-being.

- ☐ Endorphins (The Natural Painkiller): Endorphins are peptides produced by the brain that act as natural pain relievers. Often released during physical activities like exercise, laughter, or even when in pain, they help alleviate stress and promote a sense of euphoria. In the real world, this well-known 'runner's high' enhances our moods and reduces feelings of discomfort, creating a positive environment for mental health.

The Bootylicious System

- ☐ Dopamine (The Feel-Good Neurotransmitter):
  Dopamine is often referred to as the 'feel-good' hormone due to its role in the brain's reward system. It helps drive motivation and feelings of pleasure, reinforcing activities that bring us joy or satisfaction. Engaging in hobbies, achieving personal goals, or simply indulging in your favorite foods can trigger dopamine release. This powerful neurotransmitter plays a vital part in our ability to experience joy and fulfillment in life.

- ☐ Serotonin (The Mood Regulator): Serotonin is a critical hormone responsible for mood balancing. It helps regulate various functions in the body, including mood, appetite, sleep, and digestion. Higher levels of serotonin are linked to improved mood and a sense of contentment. Activities that contribute to serotonin production include exposure to sunlight, regular exercise, and a diet rich in healthy carbohydrates. Since serotonin also impacts sleep, ensuring quality rest is a significant aspect of maintaining its balance.

- ☐ Oxytocin (The Love Hormone): Oxytocin is referred to as the ultimate 'Love Hormone, which is essential for social bonding and emotional connection. In simplicity, it is released during moments of intimacy, such as hugging, touching, kissing, or childbirth, forming social bonds and building relationships. Engaging in acts of kindness, whether through volunteering, helping, serving, or simply spending time with loved ones, can stimulate the release of oxytocin, enhancing feelings of connection, community, and togetherness.

The Bootylicious System

What if we ignore our hormones? The intricate interplay of our happy, feel-good, and love hormones cannot work on our behalf as they should. Nevertheless, in *The Bootylicious System*, we do have free will to do whatever we like; however, if we do not use them, the body will operate with the negative ones. And, due to this willful oversight on our behalf, we will become a statistic or travesty in the eyes of mankind.

Unfortunately, negating Spiritual Principles and Etiquette has become a phenomenal racketeering money-making empire, capitalizing on our naivety. How so? Processed foods are high in sugar, unhealthy fats, and calories, contributing to the cycle of obesity; therefore, we must limit their consumption. To be clear, it is not that we cannot have them from time to time; it is just that we must exhibit self-control, which is one of the Fruits of the Spirit.

Our body will naturally heal itself if we do not overload it with bad stuff consistently. For example, in the *Bootylicious Plan*, we pride ourselves on using the 80/20 rule...we must eat clean 80% of the time, leaving the 20% splurges for the weekend and within certain time frames. What makes this method so important? First, the body will naturally get rid of the junk. Secondly, it prevents binging or purging while keeping the stress hormones at bay. Thirdly, it allows us to reward ourselves for eating clean 80% of the time. Nevertheless, we will discuss this plan a little later.

In the Eye of God, our bad eating habits, unwise choices, food toxins, and parasitic overloads are really making people sick and causing:

- ☐ Obesity.
- ☐ Type 2 Diabetes.
- ☐ Hypertension (High Blood Pressure).
- ☐ Cardiovascular Diseases.

- ☐ Gastrointestinal Disorders.
- ☐ Inflammation.
- ☐ Food Allergies or Intolerances.
- ☐ Chronic Fatigue Syndrome.
- ☐ Nutritional Deficiencies.
- ☐ Skin Conditions.
- ☐ Autoimmune Disorders.
- ☐ Mental Health Issues (Anxiety and Depression).
- ☐ Liver Disease.
- ☐ Kidney Disorders.
- ☐ Hormonal Imbalances.
- ☐ Malabsorption Syndromes.
- ☐ Neurological Disorders (Migraines).
- ☐ Digestive Infections (caused by parasites).
- ☐ Chronic Inflammation.
- ☐ Poor Immune Function.

Most often, we gain weight because we are secretly depressed, suppressed, oppressed, or yoked by something or someone. If we dare to own our truth, we can overcome the barriers of our issues, directly or indirectly related to our weight gain.

In all transparency, overweight individuals are not the only ones with issues! Regardless of the size of the individual, we all have issues; besides, most thin people secretly feel overweight anyway due to their mindsets, insecurities, fear of gaining weight, and negative belief systems. Really? Yes, really!

Nonetheless, for the purpose of this book, we are dealing with the what, when, where, how, and why of weight loss, weight gain, the Do-It-Yourself healthy lifestyle, how to eat clean, and how to keep the weight off, while reclaiming the *Bootylicious Queen's* Crown of Greatness.

The Bootylicious System

A Queen's Branding

In *A Queen's Branding*, let us talk about *Symbols* for a minute. *Symbols are* comprised of a lot of hidden secrets that have yet to be discovered. In my opinion, *Symbols are* an Iconic System that goes overlooked day in and day out. Yet, the *Bootylicious Queens* go unrecognized for their contributions to civilization, as well as their secrets to staying lean, fit, and powerful.

Of course, you do not need me to tell you that *Symbols* are legendary. They are all over the place; most often under the pseudonyms called LOGOS or BRANDINGS. If you overlook the fact that you are legendary in your own right, you will automatically lose your inner power or your brand. Once this happens, regardless of the size of your body, you will never feel happy or satisfied with yourself. It does not matter how much you pretend; your inner man and your actions, reactions, thoughts, beliefs, words, desires, habits, and mindset will tell the story.

Have you ever seen a person who is a size 5 think that they are fat, or a woman who is a size 16 who is so confident? The moral to the question is that everyone has a natural set point, meaning our bone structure tells us our designed body frame. If you lose your inner power or confidence, you cannot experience true happiness. You will always find something wrong or something to complain about. When you do not allow joy to reside in the depths of your soul, it becomes extremely hard to experience happiness, joy, or gratefulness simultaneously. Then again, if you do, it is fleeting, similar to getting a quick fix or a little quicky. Once that moment is over, it will drop you like a bad habit!

The Bootylicious Body: As It Pleases God® contains a powerhouse of Divine Wisdom, hints, tips, and tricks on dieting or managing your weight to establish your unique brand that is already hidden within your loins. All that is required is a willingness to listen, learn, grow, experience, experiment, document, and a commitment.

The Bootylicious Body requires that you plan, stick to the timetable, and eat certain types of food every three hours to stabilize your metabolism, keeping your energy levels consistent throughout the day. In addition, this method prevents the dreaded energy crashes that can lead to unplanned snacking or overeating later on due to skipping meals unless you are on a fast.

If you are not willing to follow these simple rules, then this *Bootylicious System* may not be the plan for you. Why not? Achieving this look of *Divine Poshness*, *As It Pleases God* with *A Queen's Brand*, is not just about luck or genetics; you must put in the work, Spiritually Tilling your own ground.

When developing the Mind, Body, Soul, and Spirit according to the Heavenly of Heavens, it requires diligence, planning, and commitment to a structured routine of workouts, nutrition, rest days, and becoming a good steward of your well-being. How does all of this work together? When we feel good, think right, behave positively, and operate with a sense of purpose and rationale, we will make better choices in our selection of foods, incorporating lean proteins, healthy fats, and fiber-rich carbohydrates. By following instructions, you will not feel hungry; in fact, you may get tired of eating or have to remind yourself to eat.

The goal is to share information on how the bush or herbal remedies work on your behalf if you will allow yourself to understand the power of eating the right foods for your body type. The point, in fact, is that if you do not feed your body accurately and regularly, your body will go into what is called starvation mode. This is when your body begins to store food, holding onto the fat rather than burning it. In all simplicity,

The Bootylicious System

your body will burn muscle rather than fat, creating a famine in your bodily functions and making your hormones go wild.

Now, on the other hand, weight loss is the direct result of burning more calories than you consume. It does not matter how many or how few carbs you enjoy or deny yourself during the day. If, at the end of your eating ventures, you have consumed a few thousand calories too many for your body type or metabolism, you will gain weight. Therefore, you must get a Dietal System in place and work it!

Also, in the *Queen's Branding* as a *Bootylicious Queen*, posh etiquette is of great importance, especially in the realm where personal branding, confidence, and charisma are essential. More importantly, when it comes to embodying the essence of a *Bootylicious Queen*, one cannot overlook the needed charactorial traits representing Christlike Behavior based on the Fruits of the Spirit.

Why do we need Christlike Etiquette as Believers? As a *Bootylicious Queen*, the way you carry yourself speaks volumes about your confidence and self-worth. Frankly, this is not to please others; it is about representing the Kingdom of God in Earthen Vessel.

Here are a few etiquette tips to enhance your *Bootylicious Branding* and System of Conveyance, but not limited to such:

- ☐ Dress for Success: Choose outfits that flatter your figure and highlight your best features while maintaining elegance.

- ☐ Posture Perfect: Stand tall and confident. Good posture enhances your elegance.

- ☐ Mind Your Manners: Always say PLEASE, EXCUSE ME, and THANK YOU. Politeness goes a long way.

The Bootylicious System

- ☐ Table Etiquette: Familiarize yourself with proper dining etiquette, including which utensils to use and how to hold your glass.

- ☐ Engage in Conversation: Listen attentively and engage in meaningful conversations without dominating the discussion.

- ☐ Avoid Slang: Use proper language and avoid slang in formal settings to sound sophisticated.

- ☐ Dress Code Awareness: Be well-versed in different dress codes (casual, business, cocktail, etc.) and adhere to them.

- ☐ Smile Often: A genuine smile can brighten your appearance and make you more approachable.

- ☐ Personal Grooming: Maintain impeccable grooming standards. This includes hair, nails, and skincare.

- ☐ Be Gracious: Accept compliments graciously while saying, 'Thank You' and make direct eye contact.

- ☐ Respect Personal Space: Be mindful of others' personal space, especially in social gatherings.

- ☐ Know When to Applaud: Clap only during appropriate moments, such as after a performance, and avoid excessive noise.

- ☐ Social Media Savvy: Your **Digital Decorum** is of great importance, so be mindful of what you post online.

The Bootylicious System

Maintain a classy and respectful online presence, even if you do not have likes or followers. Curate your social media presence to reflect your *Bootylicious Brand*, sharing content that showcases your personality and passions. Engage positively with your followers, and remember to practice good digital etiquette by respecting the privacy of others while engaging in civilized dissertations if necessary.

- ☐ Stay Sober: Know your limits when it comes to alcohol and maintain composure in social settings.

- ☐ Use Fragrance Wisely: Choose a subtle scent, as overwhelming fragrances can be repulsive.

- ☐ Gift Giving: When presenting a gift, wrap it beautifully, and include a heartfelt note.

- ☐ Network Gracefully: Engage with others at social events without being overly assertive or aggressive.

- ☐ Be Punctual: Arriving on time is a sign of respect for others' time and sets a professional tone.

- ☐ Dress Appropriately for the Occasion: Choose outfits that suit the event while remaining true to your style.

- ☐ Avoid Gossip: Steer clear of gossip and negative talk about others to maintain a positive atmosphere.

- ☐ Communicate Clearly: Speak clearly and articulate your thoughts to convey confidence.

The Bootylicious System

- ☐ Maintain Eye Contact: This shows you are engaged and interested in the conversation.

- ☐ Be an Active Listener: Nod and respond appropriately to show you value what others are saying.

- ☐ Put Your Phone Away: During gatherings, keep your phone on silent and away to avoid distractions.

- ☐ Practice Good Hygiene: A clean and fresh appearance is essential. Regularly freshen up as needed.

- ☐ Offer Help: If you see someone in need at an event, offer assistance graciously.

- ☐ Be Respectful to Service Staff: Treat servers and service personnel with kindness and respect.

- ☐ Choose Your Words Wisely: Avoid using offensive language or making inappropriate jokes.

- ☐ Stay Calm Under Pressure: Keep your composure in stressful situations to showcase your sophistication.

- ☐ Mind Your Volume: Keep your voice at a moderate volume, whether in conversation or laughter.

- ☐ Be Well-Informed: Stay updated on current events and cultural topics to engage in thoughtful discussions.

- ☐ Limit Selfies in Public: Do not overdo it on selfies, especially in formal environments.

The Bootylicious System

- ☐ Avoid Overly Tight Clothing: Choose clothes that highlight your body without compromising comfort or taste.

- ☐ Respect Differences: Embrace diversity and be open-minded in discussions about various topics.

- ☐ Know Your Audience: Tailor your conversation topics and tone according to the company you are in.

- ☐ Practice Gratitude: Express appreciation to those who support and uplift you.

- ☐ Read the Room: Be aware of the mood and dynamics within a social gathering and adapt accordingly.

- ☐ Travel Smartly: When in unfamiliar places, respect local customs and traditions.

- ☐ Know When to Leave: Recognize when it is time to gracefully exit a conversation or gathering.

- ☐ Keep an Open Mind: Be approachable to new ideas and differing opinions.

- ☐ Avoid Bragging: Share your accomplishments humbly without overshadowing others.

- ☐ Dress Modestly When Needed: In certain circumstances, such as religious sites or formal events, opt for more modest attire.

The Bootylicious System

- ☐ Celebrate Others' Success: Be genuinely happy for the achievements of others, showcasing your grace.

- ☐ Practice Self-Control: Keep your emotions in check, especially in stressful or challenging social situations.

- ☐ Stay True to Yourself: Ultimately, confidence comes from being authentic and comfortable in your own skin.

Incorporating posh etiquette into your *Bootylicious Branding* creates an unforgettable impression that goes beyond mere appearance. It is about embodying the Qualities of A Queen: eloquence, confidence, charm, and respectfulness. Adopting these etiquette tips will not only enhance your branding but also empower you to convey your true self with grace and poise, becoming the Crème de la Crème. Embrace your inner QUEEN, and let your *Bootylicious Spirit* shine brightly!

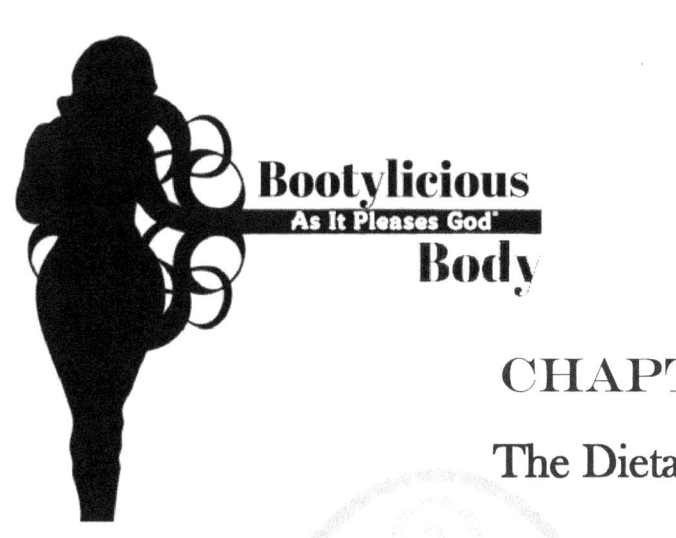

CHAPTER 3
The Dietal System

In a world where new dietary trends often lead to temporary results, disillusionment, and money grabs, *The Bootylicious Body: As It Pleases God*® paves a different path for the Kingdom. When dealing with a personalized *Dietal System* for the *Bootylicious Queens*, we take a Spiritual Approach to health and wellness, changing lives for the better. While, at the same time, bringing the *Bootylicious Queens* in Purpose on purpose to make healthier choices without the burden of restrictions violating the Spiritual Compass of free will or the fear of failure.

When we first encounter a new system in the realm of dieting and nutrition, it often feels overwhelming due to a multitude of options and conflicting information. Then again, the introduction of complex rules, guidelines, and strategies can really put the psyche of mankind on edge with hormonal imbalances, making us feel like we are embarking on a taxing journey. Yes, a journey that complicates our lives further, leaving us more confused and frustrated, rather than simplifying our lives for the Greater Good and balancing our hormones.

Whereas the introduction of *The Bootylicious Body: As It Pleases God*® aims to change this narrative. This innovative *Dietal System* is designed to cut through the confusion and make the journey to health and wellness not just straightforward but enjoyable, empowering, simple, understandable, and usable with a Spiritual Approach.

Often enough, we try to avoid the word diet due to the fear of failure, restrictions, sacrifices, and frustrations. However, once we change our perception of a diet, then we are better able to overcome the dieting woes with a mindset of wellness, wholeness, and balance.

Of course, some people insist, 'Diets do not work!' From my perspective, it is not that the diet does not work; it is that the perception of the *Dietal System* does not work for them, or there is a misalignment or misunderstanding involved in the dietal equation. For this reason, the Divine Core of *The Bootylicious Body System* is its commitment to simplicity in Earthen Vessel.

Unlike traditional diet plans that may bombard you with intricate meal plans, calorie counts, and restrictive rules, *The Bootylicious Body: As It Pleases God*® System promotes an approach that is clear with user-friendly choices. In all simplicity, we do not tell you what to eat or what to avoid; we provide the 'why' behind these choices from a Divine Perspective.

The motto for *The Bootylicious Body: As It Pleases God*® *Dietal System* is, 'You have to want it for yourself!' By allowing the psyche to participate in the choices of foods being consumed, it will not want to rebel as much, especially when using the 80/20 Rule System of consumption. We have found that breaking down the components of healthy eating into easily digestible concepts, strategies, and timings encourages a more

The Dietal System

natural and intuitive relationship with food. Plus, with this approach, it is less likely to fall upon deaf ears, especially when dealing with varying personal choices, religious preferences, and cultural backgrounds.

According to the Heavenly of Heavens, our *Dietal Systems* must be tailored to our unique lifestyles, budgets, preferences, psychological stances, and physiological needs with a little flexibility for sustainable success. If not, the strict rules may invoke the psyche to rebel against us due to feelings of guilt, restrictions, punishment, and deprivation.

Once we totally understand our *Dietal System* in real-life situations and redefine our relationship with food, we are better able to control our desire to give up or shift our responsibilities. With a mindset focused on the Temple of God instead of just a body of our own, it gives us the upper hand in our Heaven on Earth Experiences. How so? Once we master our *Dietal System* to *As It Pleases God* from selfishly pleasing ourselves, we can easily adjust our lifestyles accordingly to include success Mentally, Physically, Emotionally, and Spiritually.

A healthy lifestyle, healthy mindset, healthy eating, healthy fitness, and healthy goals are all a part of our discipline. Although eating is an addiction for some, but we cannot stop eating! We must learn what to eat, whether we have an addiction or not. In the Eye of God, being addicted to food is not totally bad for us; it is being addicted to the wrong choices of foods that are bad. Eating the right foods will naturally curb the desire to abuse food. If we do not understand what certain foods do for us, we will miss the mark and keep eating to create further damage to ourselves without realizing it.

In an era where health and dietary trends dominate our conversations, social media, and relationships, it is essential to return to a fundamental truth: We must eat to survive. As

The Dietal System

we all know, going without food, fueling the body, will begin to shut down our bodily functions. I totally understand that in our fast-paced lives, it is easy to overlook the importance of nutrition in a microwave, instant-everything society. For this reason, we must develop *The System* that works for us. If not, we will experience a wide range of negative effects, leading to serious health issues, including obesity, diabetes, heart disease, weakened immune function, muscle loss, and cognitive decline. For this reason, we must:

- ☐ Assess our health status.
- ☐ Assess our needs, goals, or desires.
- ☐ Determine the calories and nutrients required.
- ☐ Evaluate our daily routine.
- ☐ Determine the level of physical activity needed.
- ☐ Assess our current energy levels.
- ☐ Plan our meals.
- ☐ Eat slowly.
- ☐ Listen to our body.
- ☐ Stay hydrated.
- ☐ Limit caffeine and sugar intake.
- ☐ Establish a consistent sleep schedule.
- ☐ Set boundaries.
- ☐ Evaluate our work-life balance.
- ☐ Journal daily.

By becoming consciously aware of these items daily, we can indeed change the trajectory of our lives positively. Beyond a shadow of a doubt, this knowledge will empower us to adapt to *The System* of our own choosing while fostering a sense of ownership over our well-being Mentally, Physically, Emotionally, and Spiritually.

The Dietal System

The Approach

I must admit, *The Bootylicious Body* is taking the world by storm because we believe in results from the inside out, emphasizing a Spiritual Approach to health and wellness, *As It Pleases God.* This innovative *Bootylicious Program* recognizes the importance of Mental, Physical, Emotional, and Spiritual inclusion, appealing to those who seek lasting change rather than temporary solutions or quick fixes.

At the core of *The Bootylicious Body* philosophy is the understanding that various internal factors, including our mindsets, systems, nutrition, and lifestyle choices, are designed to influence building a positive relationship with every aspect of our being. More importantly, we understand that true transformation begins from within the depths of the soul, transcending the scales and mirrors. Instead, with our Divine System, established from the Heavenly of Heavens, we focus on empowerment, community, and lasting change.

Even if you have failed on other diets, the Divine Cornerstone of our nutritional educational system is designed to help you succeed. This book is not just about a diet, diet, diet! It is about education...it is about your health...it is about your livelihood...and, most of all, it is about becoming one with how you were created in the first place.

The genetic makeup that we are predicated on is a SYSTEM! For example, we all have a digestive system, cardiovascular system, skeletal system, muscular system, respiratory system, nervous system, endocrine system, immune system, reproductive system, integumentary system, and urinary system. Do you think for a minute that you can achieve an authentic Bootylicious Status without a system? If you do, it may very well affect the homeostasis (the stable regulation or equilibrium) of the other systems in your body that are designed to keep you alive and well.

The Dietal System

How do the other bodily systems affect us, especially when we know nothing about homeostasis? Regardless of whether we are in the know or not, our body is designed to heal itself through the process of homeostasis, which is crucial for survival, allowing the body to function effectively, adapt to stressors, restore balance, and maintain healthiness on our behalf. For example, homeostasis assists in temperature regulation, balancing water and electrolytes, regulating our pH balance, regulating our blood sugar through hormones like insulin and glucagon, regulating our blood pressure to ensure adequate blood flow to our organs, and maintaining our oxygen levels based on our cellular demands.

According to God's Divine Handiwork, homeostasis is intricately linked to our hormones and the psyche. If they are out of whack, it will affect the Mind, Body, Soul, and Spirit until balance is restored. For this reason, prayer, meditation, forgiveness, mercy, the use of the Fruits of the Spirit, and behaving Christlike are needed to jumpstart the homeostasis process and the regulation of our hormones properly.

In the same way that God has Divine Messengers, our hormones, senses, conscience, and instincts are our messengers for our Heaven on Earth Experiences. Now, if we choose not to use them, *As It Pleases God*, then the ramifications can deeply affect our Mental, Physical, Emotional, and Spiritual health, prompting us to self-correct, self-adjust, or self-destruct. Really? Yes, really!

Picturesquely, we often experience the longing, tugging, or turmoil within the psyche, failing to recognize what it is or what is happening. As a result, we attempt to drown it out with something or someone. Still, to no avail, it comes back like a thief in the night, descending us into a state of chaos and disarray from the inside out. Unfortunately, this imbalance can lead to various issues, including obesity, anxiety disorders, depression, insomnia, and chronic diseases,

The Dietal System

especially when unforgiveness, debauchery, and hatefulness are involved. In addition, it also has ties to jealousy, envy, pride, greed, pompousness, coveting, ungratefulness, and competitiveness. If we do not learn how to counteract these negative attributes with positive ones, using the Fruits of the Spirit, *The Imbalance* will remain.

Strike A Balance

How can an imbalance within the body remain without our permission? The psyche is an integral part of the body, regardless of whether we understand it, know about it, or ignore it...it makes its mark, doing what God designed it to do. What is that? Push us back to Him, *Spirit to Spirit*. The moment we participate in negativity, if it is not counteracted with positivity or repentance, we permit it. According to the Heavenly of Heavens, regardless of how things appear to the naked eye, if it is negative, bad, evil, unjust, or debauched, we have the right to cancel, reverse, and replace it with the appropriate scripture, positive action, or positive affirmation.

Moreover, this Spiritual Principle is also applicable to fear. Why is fear a problem for us? Fear is not technically a problem; it is designed to protect us from danger, triggering the fight-or-flight response. Then again, it can also prompt growth, awareness, red flags, or Spiritual Insight.

On the other hand, it is the constant triggering of fear that becomes the problem for us. How so? One of the biological consequences of fear is the release of cortisol, a hormone that, when elevated consistently, can have detrimental effects on our Mental, Physical, Emotional, and Spiritual Health and Well-being. If we are not formally trained to counteract the cortisol released into our systems, we can become bystanders or victims of its effects. If we do not counteract it with positivity, relaxation, or prayer, developing a positive relationship with our fears, it can taint our views, thoughts, beliefs, decisions, and food choices.

If we have a fear of eating, then we must develop a healthier way of viewing food. In my opinion, diets do not have anything to do with how we view food. We do not need a diet plan to tell us what foods are good or bad for us; we already know. We need diets to help develop discipline.

In order to have real success with any form of diet, we must change our lifestyles. Most of us think that animal protein and whole grains are the cornerstones of a healthy lifestyle; however, it is NOT. It is fruits, vegetables, and nuts! Back in ancient times, grains were used as a way to prevent families from famine, and were not to be used as a lifestyle food. Therefore, if we cut back on grains and implement more fruits, vegetables, and nuts, we will find that our bodies change and sicknesses will leave, reducing inflammation.

Keep in mind, just because someone is thin, it does not mean that they are healthy! Mismanaged and misdirected calories put on weight or cause sickness and disease, regardless of what diet we are on or our body size. An active fitness regimen is as essential to successful weight loss as cutting calories; nonetheless, in the case of your *Bootyliciousness*, cutting back on the simple carbohydrates and animal protein is ideal for the precision of your curves.

What is the purpose of cutting back on carbohydrates and animal protein? First, beyond aesthetic appeal, our curves have long been celebrated in various cultures, representing femininity, strength, and confidence. Therefore, the right balance of nutrients is required to preserve our Divine Legacy and maintain the most sought-after *Bootyliciousness*.

Secondly, not all carbohydrates are created equal. Simple carbohydrates that are found in sugary snacks, white bread, pasta, and other processed foods can lead to weight gain or

The Dietal System

diabetes and may not provide sustained energy levels, especially when combined with animal protein. On the other hand, complex carbohydrates that are found in whole grains, vegetables, and legumes can provide the necessary energy to fuel workouts and daily activities with a small amount of protein source for muscle building and satiety.

While protein is necessary for muscle repair and growth, an excess can lead to muscle gain, which does not align with the goal of achieving a softer, poshed, and more rounded *Bootyliciousness* appearance. However, if more protein is needed, plant-based protein sources, such as legumes, nuts, and seeds, can provide more of the desired nutrients and support muscle without the excess calories and hormonal imbalances that often come with animal products.

In refining your curves, *As It Pleases God*, it is also essential to incorporate more healthy fats, fiber-rich foods, and a variety of fruits and vegetables into your *Dietal System* with the mindset of quality over quantity.

The key to *The Bootylicious Body: As It Pleases God*® is to *Strike A Balance* between our nutritional intake and hormones. Does it make a difference? Absolutely. If our hormonal balance is off, the body will release other hormones to attempt to counteract the imbalance. More importantly, once this happens, something else is affected within the body. Unfortunately, our something else is not set in stone, nor is it predictable. The imbalance will target where we are the weakest, regardless of whether we understand it or not.

To redefine what it means to be the *Bootylicious Queen*, we must remain proactive to ensure that the least amount of Cortisol is released into the body. Ultimately, no one can do this for us besides the person dwelling in the body that God has BLESSED to steward.

The Dietal System

The *Bootylicious Body Dietal System* is designed to bring about an awareness of how we were created from the Beginning. When it comes to living a long and healthy life, it becomes increasingly clear that three fundamental components stand out about the secrets of longevity: we need the right foods, adequate hydration, and regular physical movement. According to the Divine Plan of God, these are the vital three ingredients for us in Earthen Vessels. Although there are more, these are the major ones that are the most beneficial for the nourishment of the Body, Mind, Soul, and Spirit.

Why are food, water, and movement the most important in the Eye of God? They bring the most balance to the body, sustaining it longer than any other components and luxuries of life. Picturesquely, look at it like this: We can eat healthily, but if we lack movement in our bodies, it breaks down by default. If we workout and move our bodies faithfully but consume the wrong foods, it breaks down by default, causing unnecessary sicknesses, inflammation, and illnesses. If we exercise and eat right but do not drink water, our bodies will break down by default, causing our blood to become thick and gooey.

Hydration Matters

Our bodies are made of mostly water, the Essence of Life, and the vital foundation of our biological existence. We are made of about 60% water. However, it can vary on a sliding scale depending on our age, sex, and hydration level. Regardless of where we are in life or what we have going on, we need water to keep our organs working properly and balance our hormones.

It does not matter how healthy or fit we are; if we lack water, we shorten our lifespan because our bodies are not able to break down food properly, transport nutrients and oxygen

The Dietal System

to cells, regulate our temperatures, participate in the cellular processes, lubricate joints, and remove or filter waste products properly through the kidneys. To avoid the buildup of toxins in our bodies, we must *Strike a Balance* in this area to ensure we safeguard our vital organs and avoid dehydration.

When it is all said and done, *Hydration Matters*. Unbeknown to most, when the body is dehydrated, our hormone levels can be disrupted, leading to various health issues, mood swings, unhealthy food cravings, and a slew of behavioral challenges. Here are the key hormones that are affected, but not limited to such:

- ☐ Antidiuretic Hormone (ADH): This hormone helps the body retain water by signaling the kidneys to conserve water instead of excreting it in urine. When hydration levels are low, ADH levels rise, which may lead to increased water retention and concentration of urine. However, chronic dehydration can hamper ADH's effectiveness, leading to imbalances.

- ☐ Cortisol: Known as the stress hormone, cortisol levels can rise in response to dehydration. Elevated cortisol levels can trigger a stress response in the body, leading to issues like anxiety and weight gain, particularly during times of chronic dehydration.

- ☐ Insulin: Proper hydration is crucial for maintaining insulin sensitivity. Dehydration can lead to insulin resistance, meaning the body does not respond effectively to insulin, which can increase the risk of type 2 diabetes. Adequate water intake helps facilitate glucose metabolism and regulates blood sugar levels.

The Dietal System

- Thyroid Hormones: The thyroid gland produces hormones that regulate metabolism, and adequate hydration is essential for optimal thyroid function. Dehydration can affect the release of thyroid hormones, leading to metabolic slowdowns and weight management difficulties.

- Sex Hormones: Water plays a role in the synthesis of sex hormones, such as estrogen and testosterone. Dehydration can lead to altered hormonal balance, potentially impacting reproductive health, libido, and overall well-being.

Regardless of whether we are new or seasoned pros, understanding the impact of hydration on hormonal balance underscores the importance of maintaining proper water intake for overall well-being. In Earthen Vessel, by prioritizing hydration, we can promote better hormonal function, enhance our Mental, Physical, Emotional, and Spiritual Well-being, and lead a healthier, more balanced life. In The *Bootylicious Body Dietal* System, to maintain optimal hydration, here are a few tips:

- Start your day with warm or room-temperature water. Drinking a glass of water first thing in the morning helps kickstart your metabolism and rehydrate after sleep.

- Drink at least eight 8-ounce glasses of water a day, but individual needs may vary based on activity level, climate, and overall health.

The Dietal System

- [ ] Include water-rich foods in your diet, such as fruits and vegetables, to enhance hydration. (cucumbers, watermelon, and oranges).

- [ ] Monitor your body for signs of dehydration, such as dry mouth, dark urine, and fatigue. A light yellow color typically indicates proper hydration, while darker urine may signify the need for more fluids.

- [ ] Set reminders. Use apps or alarms on your phone to remind you to drink water at regular intervals.

- [ ] Drink before, during, and after exercise. Staying hydrated is crucial during physical activity to maintain performance and prevent fatigue.

- [ ] After intense exercise or in hot weather, consider drinks with electrolytes (sodium, potassium, calcium) for better hydration, which are critical for nerve function and signaling.

- [ ] Limit Diuretics. Reduce intake of caffeine and alcohol, as they can lead to increased urination and dehydration.

- [ ] Infuse your water with fruits, herbs, or vegetables to enhance flavor and make it more appealing.

- [ ] Limit salty snacks. Then again, if consuming salty foods or salty snacks, always pair them with an adequate amount of hydration.

The Dietal System

- ☐ Drink non-caffeinated herbal teas. These teas can contribute to your daily hydration goals.

- ☐ Limit sugary drinks. Soft drinks and sugary juices can contribute to dehydration, so opt for water or low-calorie options instead.

- ☐ Drink an 8 oz. cup of warm water or tea before meals to aid digestion and control appetite.

- ☐ Pay attention to signs of dehydration, such as dry mouth, fatigue, or headache, and drink water accordingly.

- ☐ Remember, every sip of water counts!

Make Fitness Fun

In the ever-evolving world of the information age, the one key player in our health is a hormone called cortisol, produced by the adrenal glands, and is often referred to as the 'Stress Hormone.' When we experience stress, pressure, or disappointment, whether Mentally, Physically, Emotionally, Spiritually, Financially, or Environmentally, our bodies release cortisol by default. While this release is a natural occurrence for all mankind, the excessive release of this hormone will, once again, cause health issues, including weight gain, disrupted sleep, anxiety, a weakened immune system, and a lack of self-worth.

Exercise has been shown to reduce cortisol levels while boosting endorphins, the body's natural mood lifters, enhancing physical health, mental clarity, and emotional resilience. In addition, developing a *Spirit to Spirit* Relationship

The Dietal System

with our Heavenly Father will also help us foster a sense of peace, purpose, passion, and a sense of belonging.

In becoming good stewards of the Mind, Body, Soul, and Spirit, *As It Pleases God*, it requires active participation on our behalf. To embrace our inner *Bootylicious Queen*, we must learn to listen to our bodily needs, understand our emotions, and engage in things that promote Spiritual Health and Well-being, *As It Pleases God*.

The Bootylicious Body advocates realistic fitness goals, dropping unwanted pounds, eating new healthy foods, and being happy in the skin you are in. A great place to start this diet is with a decision to use the herbal method for supplemental nutrition, a decision to change your way of eating by using a systematic method, a decision to change the way you see food, a decision to change your attitude toward your health, and a decision to get your body moving.

When you make fitness fun, it keeps you motivated. If you find yourself bored with exercise, change your routine. You must find what you like doing; you do not have to exercise as normal people do. Simply find what works for you to keep your body moving for a certain amount of time. Listed below are a few examples of how to *Make Fitness Fun*, but not limited to such:

- ☐ Join a Group Class: Try Zumba, kickboxing, or spinning to make workouts social and fun.

- ☐ Play a Sport: Engage in basketball, soccer, or tennis to get your fitness in while enjoying some friendly competition.

The Dietal System

- ☐ Dance It Out: Put on your favorite music and dance in your living room, bedroom, patio, or take a dance class to learn some new moves.

- ☐ Go for a Hike: Explore nature trails...natural fresh air and the scenery can make hiking an enjoyable workout.

- ☐ Try a New Activity: Experiment with skating, rock climbing, paddleboarding, hula hooping, martial arts, or treasure hunting to keep things fresh and exciting.

- ☐ Set Challenges: Create personal fitness challenges or join online ones with friends to stay motivated, relevant, and accountable.

- ☐ Use Fitness Games: Play video games that require physical movement, like virtual reality games or dance games.

- ☐ Take a Scenic Bike Ride: Enjoy a leisurely bike ride through picturesque areas rather than just hitting the gym.

- ☐ Incorporate Pets: Take your dog for a run or play fetch in the park to combine fitness with quality time.

- ☐ Host a Fitness Party: Invite friends over for a group workout or an outdoor sports day for fun in a social setting.

- ☐ Change Up Your Routine: Keep your workouts varied by rotating activities or trying new gym equipment regularly.

The Dietal System

- ☐ Use Fitness Apps: Find interactive workouts or challenges that can add an element of fun and track your progress.

- ☐ Make it a Family Activity: Get the whole family involved with activities like biking, walking, talking, or playing games together.

- ☐ Go for a Swim: Spend time in the pool with fun water aerobics or simply splashing around.

- ☐ Try Outdoor Workouts: Explore parks or beaches, boot camps, or other fitness classes in a natural setting.

- ☐ Listen to Podcasts or Audiobooks: Keep your mind engaged during workouts by tuning into interesting audio content.

- ☐ Join a Community Event: Participate in local races, charity walks, or fun runs that often have a festive atmosphere.

- ☐ Create a Reward System: Set fitness goals and reward yourself when you reach them to stay motivated and committed.

- ☐ Find a Workout Buddy: Exercising with a friend can bring camaraderie, community, and accountability, making fitness more enjoyable.

- ☐ Create a Garden: This is a great way to understand the value of the Seedtime and Harvest Principle.

The Dietal System

☐ Practice Relaxing: Incorporate activities that combine fitness with relaxation and self-awareness.

I must say that 'The Bootylicious Body' is one of the best ways to shed those unwanted pounds without experiencing the horrible hunger pains, cravings, and guilt. If, for some reason, you fall off the bandwagon today, start over tomorrow without settling for defeat. The Bootylicious Body wants you to make steady efforts to stay on track. Your health and well-being are worth every dime and moment that you spend on them.

Diet and Exercise Wisdom
According to common standards, a healthy person often has a balanced diet, regular exercise, and positive social interactions. However, when faced with illness or disabilities, the strategies that maintain their health may not work in reverse. For example, a typical healthy lifestyle choice like a rigorous workout may be detrimental to someone recovering from illness, whose body requires rest and gentle movement rather than strenuous activity. Nor will it work for those with ailing disabilities, as preserving their lives becomes an even more necessity or urgent matter.

Diet and Exercise Wisdom is not one-size-fits-all. For some, this involves tailored treatment plans, exercise routines, or alternative therapies based on genetics, overall health, history, lifestyle, and other factors. In all reality, regardless of whether we are *Bootylicious* or not, it is crucial to support unwell individuals with sensitivity and compassion rather than prescribing solutions based on our own experiences, biases, or conditionings.

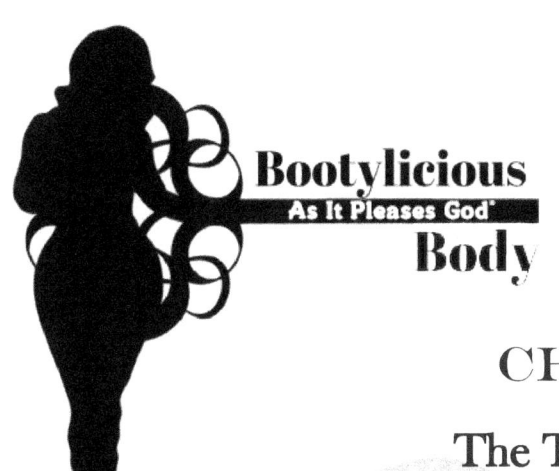

CHAPTER 4

The Temple of God

The secrets to healthily embracing your curves are already within you, *The Temple of God*. According to the Heavenly of Heavens, a significant shift is underway with your mindset and heart posture regarding your individualized self-love and self-acceptance. With a shift of perspective in this Divine Movement, understanding your body type is hidden within your self-talk and self-affirmations concerning your beauty, strength, willingness, tenacity, and health prioritization.

The celebration of diverse body types, especially curvy figures, is becoming more mainstream because God did not create everyone with the same specs. The secret to healthily embracing your curves, or the lack thereof, starts from within with a Spiritual Approach to the Mind, Body, Soul, and Spirit. Any other ways outside of this Divine Design and genetic makeup are fleeting, even if we play pretend. Without further ado, let us discuss this a little more in-depth.

The Temple of God

The Sacred Space where the Divine Presence of the Holy Trinity dwells within you, my *Bootylicious Queen*. For the Sacredness of the Holy of Holies to come alive from within, it requires a life that embodies grace, humility, obedience, purpose, and reverence with a work-in-progress mindset.

If you think *The Temple of God* is unrealistic or bogus, then please allow me to Spiritually Align this matter before going any further with *The Bootylicious Body*. 1 Corinthians 6:19-20 has a profound question and statement for you, us, and them: *"Do you not know that your body is the temple of the Holy Spirit who is in you, whom you have from God, and you are not your own? For you were bought at a price; therefore glorify God in your body and in your spirit, which are God's."*

According to the Heavenly of Heavens, to evolve into a Divine Temple, *As It Pleases* God, our lives must reflect some form of Holiness and Purity with the correct heart and mind posture. When trusting His Divine Plan, even in times of uncertainty, Holiness is not about perfection at all, as most would think. Ultimately, it is more about the intentionality in living in a state of faith, hope, and love that is conducive to Spiritual Growth, Usability, and Elevation for the Kingdom of God. While simultaneously using the Fruits of the Spirit, behaving Christlike, self-correcting along the way, and remaining a healthy and vibrant reflection of God's Divine Creation.

What does all of this mean in layman's terms? Amid all of our *Bootyliciousness* and Poshness, we must represent the Kingdom of God, Mentally, Physically, Emotionally, Spiritually, Financially, and Collectively. God frowns on us behaving waywardly, rudely, and foolishly. Why would He frown, especially when we have free will? In a world filled with choices and decisions, the way we conduct ourselves publicly and privately can significantly affect our lives and the

The Temple of God

lives of those around us. Regardless of our level of free will, we are a walking and talking billboard, and when we are dealing with *The Temple of God* in a *Bootylicious Body*, we must represent!

How do we know if we are representing the Kingdom of God or not? According to Matthew 7:20, *"By their fruits you will know them."* In all of our *Bootyliciousness*, our fruits will outdo us every time. Therefore, if we have lingering bad fruits, it is time to make them good. Conversely, if we already have good fruits, it is time to make them better and share them with others based on the Law of Reciprocity and Seedtime and Harvest.

What do fruits have to do with our *Bootylicious Body*? Suppose we do not represent sweet fruits or the Fruits of the Spirit (Love, Joy, Peace, Patience, Kindness, Goodness, Faithfulness, Gentleness, and Self-Control), *As It Pleases God*. In this case, our fruits have the potential to become bittersweet, unpalatable, or rotten at the core. Unfortunately, this happens all too often...where we have a female with an absolutely banging body, but the moment she opens her mouth, her beauty turns into all types of unpleasantries.

Before we go any further, please allow me to Spiritually Align our actions and outcomes associated with good and bad fruits, according to Matthew 7:16-19. *"You will know them by their fruits. Do men gather grapes from thornbushes or figs from thistles? Even so, every good tree bears good fruit, but a bad tree bears bad fruit. A good tree cannot bear bad fruit, nor can a bad tree bear good fruit. Every tree that does not bear good fruit is cut down and thrown into the fire."* As *Bootylicious Queens*, in the Eye of God, we are required to self-correct our negative or bad character traits and deeds into good ones.

When building strength and accountability, *As It Pleases God*, regardless of whether you perceive yourself as *Bootylicious*

The Temple of God

or bodacious, you belong to the Creator of it all. More importantly, *The Bootylicious Body* gives you the option of treating your body like a TEMPLE or a TENT. You cannot eat badly and think that you will achieve good results, even if you are thin.

As a word of caution, thin does not mean healthy! You can indeed lose weight by eating unhealthily, and you can indeed become thin by eating unhealthily as well. Nevertheless, you must take into account what is going on from within. My *Bootylicious Queen*, your inner health is the key to your authentic *Bootylicious Body*.

The bottom line is that regardless of where you are in life or how you feel, your body will need nutrients, water, and movement. In a world where fleeting trends and social media influencers attempt to dictate the Divine Standards of beauty, *The Bootylicious Body* does not promise overnight success, but it does promise results! Remember, we are all a work-in-progress, and it is going to take some time to master the system of *The Bootylicious Body: As It Pleases God*®.

From my professional perspective, the importance of dieting transcends mere weight loss; it encompasses a broader spectrum of health that includes Mental, Physical, Emotional, and Spiritual Well-Being, serving as a Divine Cornerstone or decrepit downfall. How so? Simply put, first, it can work for us if we are ready for it with a comprehensive approach. Secondly, it can also work against us if:

- ☐ We are not ready.
- ☐ We are unprepared.
- ☐ We lack diligence.
- ☐ We are uncommitted.
- ☐ We are easily distracted.
- ☐ We feel restricted.
- ☐ We feel pressured.

The Temple of God

☐ We find psychological comfort in stress eating.

Do we not all find comfort in eating? We all do to a certain extent. The goal is to respect food as nourishment and community. In the Eye of God, we should never abuse food as a pastime to block out our issues, regardless of what size we are or what the scale says.

The risks and consequences of being overweight or unhealthy are factors that we must take into consideration. Our eating habits can come from an addiction to certain types of foods, an emotional need, conditioning, cravings, learned behavior, and the list goes on.

The flip-flopping or yo-yoing dieting must come to an end. You must give yourself the opportunity to succeed at shedding pounds the right way, with the right plan, and with the right information. You can take as many shortcuts as you want; if you do, more than likely, you will find yourself starting over again until you finally get it right.

When you are busy or moving your body, you have less time to think about eating or snacking. When you sit around watching TV, the commercials are designed to make you crave food. The subliminal messaging plays a keen role in you becoming tempted to eat when you are not hungry or eat the things that you should not be eating unless it is your free day. Another pitfall when it comes to dieting is that we give up on ourselves at the first sign of defeat.

Listen, the scale can be your best friend or your worst enemy when dieting, depending upon your perception. If you weigh yourself every day, it is a possibility that you may be setting yourself up for failure. Your weight will fluctuate, and if you are determining your mood based on what the scale is saying, then you have just given your scale the power over you.

The Temple of God

Massive overnight weight loss is not possible; it takes time. Therefore, you must change your mindset for the best and most sustainable results.

The Power of Agreement

Regardless of whether we are seeking a *Bootylicious Body* or not, we are all created in the Image of God. In addition, we are all His Divine Creation, even if we do not feel as such.

According to the Heavenly of Heavens, our inherent value is expressed through us and by us. It is not expressed through a third party unless there is some form of Spiritual Intercession or Agreement occurring on our behalf. Matthew 18:19-20 says, *"Again I say to you that if two of you agree on earth concerning anything that they ask, it will be done for them by My Father in heaven. For where two or three are gathered together in My name, I am there in the midst of them."*

The significance of being a Temple of God is wrapped in our *Power of Agreement*. We can agree with God, ourselves, and others, but the most important agreement for our Heaven on Earth Experiences is to come into Divine Agreement with being *The Temple of God*, and *As It Pleases Him*.

What makes this Spiritual Agreement so powerful for Believers? Choosing to wholeheartedly please God with our Mind, Body, Soul, and Spirit gives us Kingdom Leverage that most are not privy to having, especially when becoming a work-in-progress, *As It Pleases Him*.

For example, once you come into AGREEMENT with having a *Bootylicious Body: As It Pleases God*, the Holy Spirit will begin to assist you on this Spiritual Journey if you follow the instructions placed before you. What makes me or this *Bootylicious System* so special? I came into a Spiritual

The Temple of God

Agreement with my Heavenly Father in Earthen Vessel to deliver a Divine Message to you, providing a path.

If you walk in it as instructed, it means you and I AGREE with God together for the fulfillment of the *Bootylicious Dietal System*. All of which is based on Ecclesiastes 4:9-12: *"Two are better than one, because they have a good reward for their labor. For if they fall, one will lift up his companion. But woe to him who is alone when he falls, for he has no one to help him up. Again, if two lie down together, they will keep warm; but how can one be warm alone? Though one may be overpowered by another, two can withstand him. And a threefold cord is not quickly broken."*

Temple Maintenance

In the Eye of God, to achieve, sustain, and maintain our state of *Bootyliciousness*, according to the Heavenly of Heavens, *Temple Maintenance* is mandatory for the upkeep of the Four Corners of the Mind, Body, Soul, and Spirit. Due to the lack of understanding, this is rarely spoken about from a Divine Perspective in the Spirit of Quaternity. But, for what we are attempting to accomplish here with *Temple Maintenance*, it must be unveiled.

What is the Spirit of Quaternity? When dealing with the Temple of God, it is putting the Holy Trinity (The Father, Son, and Holy Spirit) into the four essential parts of our being. To be clear, there are more aspects of our being, but the Mind, Body, Soul, and Spirit are the most important for our Heaven on Earth Experience in Earthen Vessels to bring forth Spiritual Balance, *As It Pleases God*. If we miss one of them, it will throw the core of our being off-center, affecting our genius and creative capabilities as well as our senses, conscience, and instincts.

The Temple of God

As we journey through life, we experience multiple forms of Quaternity without realizing it. In all transparency, it is nothing spooky or diabolical. Conversely, if we do not understand it, it can definitely make us feel this way, especially when the Vicissitudes and Cycles of Life decide to correct us. Here are a few ways Quaternity is right in our faces without realizing it:

- ☐ We have the Foundational Four Elements: Earth, Water, Fire, and Air.
- ☐ We have the Four Cardinal Directions: North, South, East, and West.
- ☐ We have the Four Seasons: Spring, Summer, Winter, and Fall.
- ☐ We have the Four Stages of Life: Childhood, Adolescence, Adulthood, and Old Age.
- ☐ We have the Water Cycle: Evaporation, Condensation, Precipitation, and Collection.
- ☐ We have Project Management: Initiation, Planning, Execution, and Closure.
- ☐ We have the Sales Process: Prospecting, Qualification, Presentation, and Closing.
- ☐ We have Human Gestation: First Trimester, Second Trimester, Third Trimester, and Birth.
- ☐ We have Crisis Management: Prevention, Preparation, Response, and Recovery.
- ☐ We have the Personal Growth Journey: Awareness, Acceptance, Action, and Mastery.
- ☐ We have the Process of Learning: Acquisition, Retention, Recall, and Application.
- ☐ We have the Phases of a Relationship: Attraction, Reality, Intimacy, and Commitment.
- ☐ We have the Stages of Grief: Denial, Anger, Bargaining, and Acceptance.

The Temple of God

- ☐ We have the Four Stages of Sleep: NREM Stage 1 (Light Sleep), NREM Stage 2 (Moderate Sleep), NREM Stage 3 (Deep Sleep), and REM sleep (Rapid Eye Movement Sleep).
- ☐ We have the Nutrition Cycle: Intake, Digestion, Absorption, and Elimination.

Once we perfect the Mind, Body, Soul, and Spirit, the Spiritual Quaternity hidden within everything else will work itself out. In my opinion, this is similar to when getting cut; the body jumps into action, forming clots to stop the bleeding while attempting to heal itself.

To enhance our clarity, strength, and Spiritual Fulfillment with the *Bootylicious Body's System*, we must exercise wisdom, treating our bodies as *The Temple of God* with respect, purity, and care. Regardless of how we feel, think, or behave, we are interconnected, even if we seemingly feel disconnected. The right balance of macronutrients, vitamins, and minerals not only strengthens our bodies but also nurtures our minds, allowing us to pursue our Spiritual Paths with a renewed sense of purpose.

Is *Temple Maintenance* some sort of joke? Absolutely not. How we perceive and treat our bodies matters in the Eye of God because we are indeed His Sacred Space. Here is what Paul says in 1 Corinthians 6:19-20: *"Do you not know that your body is the temple of the Holy Spirit who is in you, whom you have from God, and you are not your own? For you were bought at a price; therefore glorify God in your body and in your spirit, which are God's."*

When engaging in Spiritual Maintenance, *As It Pleases God*, we must MASTER the charactorial traits He loves while turning away from what He hates. Of course, we will always have free will to do, say, and become whatever we like with

The Temple of God

whomever. Still, it does not negate the Divine Expectations set before us or the Spiritual Etiquette required of us as *Bootylicious Queens* and Kingdom Citizens.

As a *Bootylicious Queen* myself, it is my reasonable service to activate the Law of Reciprocity on the topic that often gets swept under the rug of religiosity. First and foremost, God will move Heaven and Earth for us with Supernatural Favor when we faithfully use the Fruits of the Spirit, *As It Pleases Him*.

For the *Bootylicious Queens* that are not familiar with the Fruits of the Spirit, they are found in Galatians 5:22-23. They are:

- ☐ Love.
- ☐ Joy.
- ☐ Peace.
- ☐ Long-suffering (Patience).
- ☐ Kindness.
- ☐ Goodness.
- ☐ Faithfulness.
- ☐ Gentleness.
- ☐ Self-control.

Against such things, there is NO LAW. According to the Heavenly of Heavens, these charactorial attributes reflect the ideal life lived in accordance with the Holy Spirit and Christlikeness. In my opinion, doing a self-analysis using the Fruits of the Spirit helps us to self-correct a lot better. Here is how it works with *Temple Maintenance*: Ask yourself...

- ☐ Is it loving? Am I sharing love? Was that loving?
- ☐ Am I joyful? Do I feel joyful? Am I sharing joyfulness?
- ☐ Am I peaceful? Am I extending peace?
- ☐ Am I being patient? Have I lost my patience?

The Temple of God

- ☐ Am I being kind? Am I extending kindness to them?
- ☐ Am I sharing goodness? Am I being a good person?
- ☐ Am I being faithful? Am I representing faithfulness?
- ☐ Am I being gentle? Are my words and behaviors gentle?
- ☐ Am I exhibiting self-control? Have I lost control in this matter? How do I regain control over myself?

Suppose we do not query ourselves in such a manner. In this case, the psyche will get out of control, placing us on a rollercoaster of negativity and debauchery while appearing right in our own eyes. Without self-correction or self-mirroring, it becomes extremely challenging to participate in what God loves with the correct heart and mind posture.

Why must we go through all of these hoops just to please God? It is not for Him alone; it is for us...helping us to rightly divide good from bad, right from wrong, just from unjust, positive from negative, and so on.

The Spiritual Duality from the Garden of Eden still exists, affecting mankind to this very day; therefore, we must know the equal and opposite of our actions, thoughts, words, beliefs, desires, habits, or traumas. If not, we will fall for the okey doke easily, selling our souls to the highest bidder. For this reason, 2 Timothy 2:15 says, *"Be diligent to present yourself approved to God, a worker who does not need to be ashamed, rightly dividing the word of truth."*

Aside from the use of the Fruits of the Spirit to perfect our Spiritual Fruits in the *Temple Maintenance* Process, here are a few other things God loves, but is not limited to such:

- ☐ He Loves A Cheerful Giver. *"So let each one give as he purposes in his heart, not grudgingly or of necessity; for God loves a cheerful giver."* 2 Corinthians 9:7.

The Temple of God

- ☐ He Loves Righteousness. *"For You are not a God who takes pleasure in wickedness, nor shall evil dwell with You."* Psalm 5:4.

- ☐ He Loves Truth. *"Lying lips are an abomination to the Lord, But those who deal truthfully are His delight."* Proverbs 12:22.

- ☐ He Loves Mercy. *"For I desire mercy and not sacrifice, and the knowledge of God more than burnt offerings."* Hosea 6:6.

- ☐ He Loves Humility. *"For though the Lord is on high, yet He regards the lowly; but the proud He knows from afar."* Psalm 138:6.

- ☐ He Loves Justice. *"The Lord loves justice, and does not forsake His saints."* Psalm 37:28.

- ☐ He Loves Obedience. *"Children, obey your parents in all things, for this is well pleasing to the Lord."* Colossians 3:20.

- ☐ He Loves Gratitude. *"In everything give thanks; for this is the will of God in Christ Jesus for you."* 1 Thessalonians 5:18.

- ☐ He Loves Worship. *"God is Spirit, and those who worship Him must worship in spirit and truth."* John 4:24.

- ☐ He Loves Purity. *"Blessed are the pure in heart, for they shall see God."* Matthew 5:8.

The Temple of God

- ☐ He Loves Forgiveness. *"And be kind to one another, tenderhearted, forgiving one another, even as God in Christ forgave you."* Ephesians 4:32.
- ☐ He Loves Sinners Who Repent. *"I say to you that likewise there will be more joy in heaven over one sinner who repents than over ninety-nine just persons who need no repentance."* Luke 15:7.

- ☐ He Loves His Divine Creation. *"The earth is the Lord's, and all its fullness, the world and those who dwell therein."* Psalm 24:1.

- ☐ He Loves Unity. *"That they all may be one, as You, Father, are in Me, and I in You; that they also may be one in Us."* John 17:21.

Regardless of whether we like our *Bootyliciousness* or not, we all have options when it comes down to the *Temple of God*. In my opinion, there is no reason to have a banging body with bad character while exhibiting seditious behaviors, thoughts, beliefs, and desires. Showing out in public or private is not cute, not now and not ever!

No judgment intended; I, too, had to learn this same information with zero help from mankind. I had to seek the Lord, for real, for real! He heard my cry, and He answered me with Divine Wisdom on another LEVEL, confounding human reasoning. So, in order to feed His sheep, I am unveiling the Kingdom's Secrets in maintaining the *Bootyliciousness* and Divine Sacredness of our Forefathers.

Now, let us get to the things God hates. Some would say hate is a negative character trait...and it is! Especially when it is directed toward a person, place, or thing. Nevertheless, when it is directed toward a character trait, behavior, thought, desire, or habit, we can dislike or hate it all day long.

Here is the key: There is a difference between hating someone or something breathing the Breath of Life and hating something that does not have blood flowing through its veins or have a DNA structure.

Throughout the scriptures, Believers are called to reflect on the nature of God and His expectations, *As It Pleases Him*. Unfortunately, for some odd reason, we overlook Genesis 1:31: *"Then God saw everything that He had made, and indeed it was very good. So the evening and the morning were the sixth day."* If anything or anyone falls under the category of GOOD in the Eye of God, please do not hate on it or them.

More importantly, if you do not like yourself, then God has a problem with your unlikability. Why would He have a problem, especially when having free will? Whether you know it or not, there is good in you hidden under layers of something else. Furthermore, as a Child of God, it is your responsibility to extract it, *As It Pleases Him*, to avoid becoming or remaining Spiritually Blind, Deaf, or Mute. If not, you will find yourself in a web of disdainment, selfishly pleasing yourself. All of this will cause you to get a Spiritual Side-eye with stunted growth, publicly or privately.

Why are we penalized for not knowing the good that resides within the depths of our souls? According to the Heavenly of Heavens, certain behaviors, attitudes, and characteristics are detestable to God. Plus, if you cannot see the good in yourself, it is extremely difficult to recognize it in others, nor can you properly exhibit mercy and compassion for another without conditions. If you say that you can, then deception is waiting to deceive you further.

Why would the Spirit of Deception wait to deceive us as Believers? We all have a dual nature, even if we are Holy Ghost-Filled and Fire-Baptized. The difference between an

The Temple of God

effective and ineffective Believer is the ability to reverse, cast down, and remove the dualism effect. We all consciously or subconsciously know right from wrong, but we do not all know how to reverse or correct it, *As It Pleases God*. Instead, we make up stuff or pretend based on our own perceptions and ideologies, especially when God clearly tells us what He does not like, but we do it anyway.

Remember this: You will never have to teach a child how to do wrong; it is in their nature; however, you must teach them how to do the right thing...for it is in their nature as well.

Conversely, in Spiritual Development, if you do not know or understand what the detestable behaviors, attitudes, or characteristics are, you will 'get got' by the enemy's wiles. Thus, in the *Bootylicious Body: As It Pleases God*®, you need to know what they are to ensure your *Bootyliciousness* does not become repulsive or delusional.

According to Proverbs 6:16-19, seven things are detestable to Him:

- ☐ A proud look. (Pride).
- ☐ A lying tongue. (Dishonesty).
- ☐ Hands that shed innocent blood. (Violence/Injustice).
- ☐ A heart that devises wicked plans. (Wicked Plots).
- ☐ Feet that are swift in running to evil. (Deception).
- ☐ A false witness who speaks lies. (A Liar).
- ☐ One who sows discord among brethren. (Chaos, Division, and Confusion).

Your moral and ethical behaviors are on the Divine Radar of the Kingdom of God. If you are exhibiting any of these negative behaviors out of defiance, selfishness, or impulsivity, it is time to self-correct.

The Temple of God

Why must we self-correct, especially when we have grace? With or without grace, if you do not speak to the duality of your character, it will speak to you with or without your permission.

Unfortunately, this is where we get the negative chatter, chatting away at its own whim while dumping toxins into our minds. Now, if we do not stop it or counteract it, then who will? Since we are the only ones allowing access, then it means we have the wherewithal to bring the negativity or debauchery to a complete halt. Grace cannot do this for us; we must do it and allow grace to do its job in refining us, *As It Pleases God*.

On the other hand, if others are exhibiting these behaviors, exercise caution while using the Fruits of the Spirit in your approach or exit. Why must we get rid of them or exit? When using the Fruits of the Spirit, we do not do the pruning...God does. Nevertheless, we must become prepared Mentally, Physically, and Emotionally to let go with clean hands and a pure heart, bearing no grudges while operating in the Spirit of Excellence.

As a Word to the Wise, it is always best to allow God to pull out the pruning shears. Spiritually Speaking, we do not always know in advance what or who He is using to train, mold, prepare, teach, or test us.

Listen, while in the Spiritual Classroom, if we glean the lessons while getting an understanding, *As It Pleases God*, it carries a ton of Spiritual Weight in the Kingdom. In addition, as icing on the cake, if we use the Fruits of the Spirit and behave Christlike when doing so, no one or nothing can contend with an OBEDIENT Child of God who is about their Father's Business. In my opinion, we should never compromise on the *Temple Maintenance* needed to polish up our Spiritual Etiquette or *Bootyliciousness*.

The Temple of God

Why is *Temple Maintenance* so important in the Eye of God? Once our *Bootylicious Mindset* becomes established, *As It Pleases God*, we must possess the wherewithal to sustain it with the correct Spiritual Nutrients. Conversely, if we do not equip ourselves, *As It Pleases Him*, envy, jealousy, pride, greed, coveting, and competitiveness can place us in a Spiritual Chokehold. So, it is imperative to build the foundation of *The Temple of God* with the Spiritual Manual for its upkeep, especially when dealing with the Mind, Body, Soul, and Spirit.

What are the indications of having an issue with envy, jealousy, pride, greed, coveting, and competitiveness? Although everyone is a little different due to varying traumas, conditioning, motives, and mindsets; however, listed below are a few indicators, but not limited to such:

- ☐ Constant Comparison: If you find yourself frequently comparing yourself to others, feeling inadequate or superior based on those comparisons, or finding fault in others, there is an issue from within taking place.

- ☐ Resentment Toward Others' Success: If you feel anger, rage, hatred, or bitterness when someone else achieves something you desire, there is an issue from within taking place.

- ☐ Obsessive Thoughts: If you find yourself ruminating over what others have or what they do while wishing it were yours, there is an issue from within taking place.

- ☐ Self-Importance: If you find yourself exhibiting a sense of superiority or entitlement, believing you are better than others, there is an issue from within taking place.

The Temple of God

- ☐ Difficulty Celebrating Others: If you find yourself struggling to feel happy for friends or family members when they succeed, there is an issue from within taking place.

- ☐ Materialism: If you find yourself with an intense focus on acquiring material possessions or wealth, often at the expense of personal relationships, there is an issue from within taking place.

- ☐ Misdirected Anger: If you find yourself feeling frustrated or angry at others without understanding the root cause of that emotion, often tied to feelings of jealousy, there is an issue from within taking place.

- ☐ Coveting Others' Relationships: If you find yourself desiring what others have in terms of friendships or romantic partnerships, often leading to feelings of inadequacy, there is an issue from within taking place.

- ☐ Overcompetitive Behavior: If you find yourself constantly wanting to one-up others, even in situations where competition is unnecessary, there is an issue from within taking place.

- ☐ Discontent with Achievements: If you find yourself feeling unsatisfied with your accomplishments because you believe they do not measure up to others, there is an issue from within taking place.

- ☐ Gossip or Slander: If you find yourself speaking negatively about others to diminish their achievements or character, there is an issue from within taking place.

The Temple of God

- ☐ Strained Relationships: If you find yourself experiencing frequent conflicts, unresolved issues, or constant bouts of tension in relationships, friendships, or with family members, there is an issue from within taking place. Even if we are not the problem, the goal is to find a solution, period!

- ☐ Fear of Loss: If you find yourself fearing that others will take away what you have, whether it is relationships, success, or possessions, there is an issue from within taking place.

- ☐ Overreaction to Criticism: If you find yourself taking offense easily and reacting defensively or negatively when justifiably or unjustifiably critiqued, there is an issue from within taking place. More importantly, if you have not learned how to reverse engineer criticism from negative to positive at the drop of a dime, you have work to do.

- ☐ Inability to Apologize: If you find yourself finding it difficult to admit mistakes or say sorry due to an inflated sense of selfishness or pride, there is an issue from within taking place.

- ☐ Emotional Exhaustion: If you find yourself feeling drained from being around those who possess more than you, there is an issue from within taking place.

- ☐ Manipulative Behaviors: If you find yourself trying to undermine others to elevate your own status or success, there is an issue from within taking place.

The Temple of God

- ☐ Avoidance of Others: If you find yourself pulling away from friends or family members for fear of being judged for what you possess or do not possess, there is an issue from within taking place.

- ☐ Seeking Validation: If you find yourself constantly needing approval from others to feel good about yourself, there is an issue from within taking place.

- ☐ Ignoring Gratitude: If you find yourself focusing on what you lack instead of appreciating what you have, leading to a perpetually discontented mindset, there is an issue from within taking place.

Recognizing these signs can be the first step toward healthily addressing these feelings, thoughts, desires, and fears to combat underlying insecurities. Although we all have insecurities, but we do not all know what they are, how to deal with them, or what triggers them. Remember, as a *Temple of God* in a *Bootylicious Body*, our lives are about a Spiritual Journey of Self-Improvement and *Self-Acceptance*, taking one step at a time toward a healthier Mind, Body, Soul, and Spirit. So, let us talk about this a little more in the next chapter.

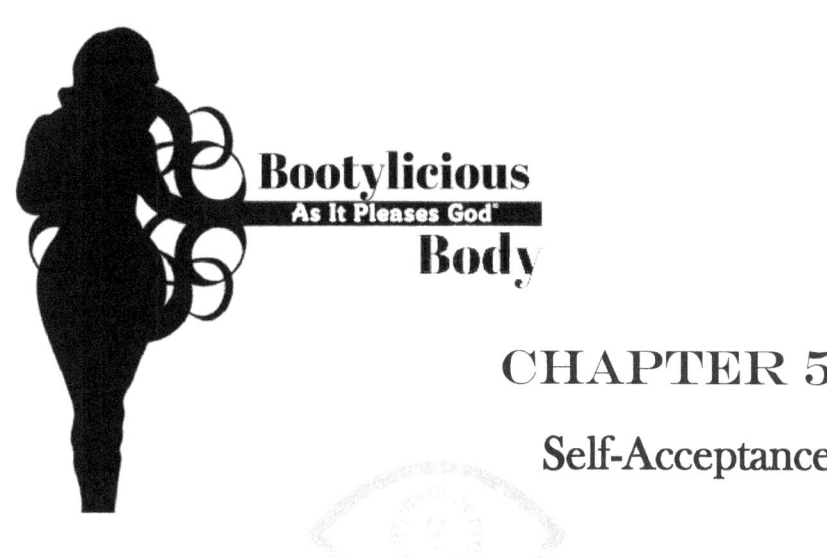

CHAPTER 5

Self-Acceptance

In a world filled with comparisons, expectations, competitiveness, standards, and social media influences, our *Bootylicious Journey* toward *Self-Acceptance* can often feel far-fetched or overwhelming when adjusting our mindsets. To elevate this feeling, we must come to terms with our strengths, weaknesses, and imperfections. Doing so helps us foster a sense of freedom and authenticity without depending on external validation.

Self-Acceptance is all about recognizing and appreciating ourselves for who we are without becoming critical, demeaning, or repulsive. At the core, selflessly loving ourselves gives us the ability to learn, grow, and handle life's challenges to love others, *As It Pleases God*.

How can we selflessly love ourselves? Selfless love involves humility, mercy, and compassion for ourselves and others. To get to this state of being, *As It Pleases God*, we must use the Fruits of the Spirit and behave Christlike. In creating a safe

Self-Acceptance

space for ourselves and others, here are a few things we need to glean from our *Bootyliciousness*, but not limited to such:

- ☐ We need an understanding of deception.
- ☐ We must challenge negativity and debauchery.
- ☐ We need to master moving forward.
- ☐ We must communicate effectively.
- ☐ We must be willing to be in Purpose on purpose.

By consciously choosing to engage with integrity and purpose, we must accept the fact that failure and setbacks are a part of life designed to help us regroup, learn, and move forward in the Spirit of Excellence. Here are a few questions to help develop our Self-Awareness, *As It Pleases God*.

- ☐ What are my current beliefs about my body and health?
- ☐ How do I define a *Bootylicious Body* for myself?
- ☐ What positive traits do I appreciate about my body?
- ☐ What specific goals do I have for my physical fitness?
- ☐ How does my daily routine support or hinder my fitness goals?
- ☐ What foods make me feel energized and healthy?
- ☐ How do I handle setbacks or challenges in my fitness journey?
- ☐ Who influences my perception of beauty and health?
- ☐ How do I feel emotionally about my body?
- ☐ What actions can I take to cultivate a more positive body image?
- ☐ Am I comparing myself to others, and how does that affect my self-image?
- ☐ What do I enjoy most about exercise and physical activity?
- ☐ How do I celebrate my achievements, big or small?

Self-Acceptance

- ☐ What role does self-compassion play in my Bootylicious Journey to *Self-Awareness*?
- ☐ How do my Spiritual Beliefs intersect with my views on health and body image?
- ☐ What practices can I implement to enhance my self-discipline?
- ☐ How do I seek support from friends and family in reaching my goals?
- ☐ In what ways can I be kinder to myself on this journey?
- ☐ What does a balanced lifestyle look like for me?
- ☐ How can I align my self-care practices with my personal values and beliefs?

Make sure your answers are properly documented in your *Bootylicious Journal* to ensure you are becoming more in tune with your true self.

Understanding Deception

When it comes to the *Bootylicious Body Experience*, according to the Heavenly of Heavens, we must deal with two things: fear and shame. These two annoying factors have privately plagued society beyond measure, and now is the time to understand the birth of shame itself. But of course, without shame, there would be no fear, right? Wrong! Fear is designed to work for us and not against us; nevertheless, once we introduce shame into the equation, it becomes the BEAST, similar to what is spoken about in the Book of Revelation.

How do we introduce a Beast into our lives when we are not beasts at all...instead, we are Believers? Unfortunately, this is how we become deceived. The picturesque view from our mind's eye paints a fairytale picture of a wild beast in the

Self-Acceptance

elements of nature that seemingly do not apply to us. Nonetheless, in the Eye of God, it is applicable, even if we are Spiritually Blind, Deaf, or Mute.

Here is what Revelation 20:10 says, *"The devil, who deceived them, was cast into the lake of fire and brimstone where the beast and the false prophet are. And they will be tormented day and night forever and ever."* Now, the question is, 'Who is the Beast, and who is the False Prophet?' Then again, 'Can the Prophet possess the Beast or the Beast possess the Prophet when deceived by the Devil?' Well, I will say this, 'God lumped them all in the same category because the Prophet or Believer should have counteracted the deceit from jump!'

The moment we think the Book of Revelation is not playing itself out from within the psyche of mankind, we are sadly mistaken. The torment is happening, and yet we pretend as if we are above reproach or that it is far-fetched. Then again, we are waiting for the Bridegroom to come, and He is already here, seating the Table, in the hope that we will awaken from our deceptive slumbers.

Why is our slumbering considered deceptive as Believers? Unfortunately, it is due to our lack of understanding, our lack of knowledge, and our outright participation in willful disobedience. Listen, we all have a good and bad side, depending on our thoughts, beliefs, traumas, triggers, and even the lies we tell ourselves that contribute to the internal Beast. To be clear and with all due respect, I am not calling anyone a Beast here. I am referring to a character trait that we all possess that adds to the complexity of our human experience in Earthen Vessels.

According to the Heavenly of Heavens, due to the little glitch in our dual nature, we must exhibit self-control to ensure we do not become out of control. Frankly, without self-control or due to the lack of understanding, the Beast that we hide will take over within our very own psyche, especially

Self-Acceptance

when disobedience and pretense are involved with our ungoverned emotions.

The moment we pretend the Beast is not there, it has already taken over with the Spirit of Deception, preventing us from discerning positive from negative, right from wrong, just from unjust, and so on, calling good evil and evil good. For this reason, as a *Bootylicious Queen*, it is wise to know our thoughts, beliefs, traumas, desires, and triggers to ensure we can plead the Blood of Jesus over them and counteract them with the Word of God.

In addition, we can also allow the Holy Spirit to tame the hidden Beast from within to prevent us from turning on ourselves when we least expect it. The bottom line is that in order to grow authentically in the Light, *As It Pleases God*, we must address the dark areas to live in balance and harmony with ourselves and others. If not, the darkness can literally haunt, yoke, challenge, and provoke us. Is this real? Absolutely. It is as real as putting on two left shoes, trying to go right while standing straight, or *Moving Forward* without appearing awkward or unbalanced! If one does not understand this whimsical analogy of discomfort, let us talk a little more about how operating in such a manner makes us unnatural and clumsy in the Eye of God. Why? Ill-fitted or two left shoes symbolize an internal conflict, especially with our interactions, values, passions, goals, and decisions in need of retrospection, growth, or change before *Moving Forward*.

Moving Forward

In order to take our *Bootylicious Bodies* forward with an understanding of our hidden intricacies, we must take a step back to the point of origin. Initially, Adam and Eve dwelled in a world devoid of shame, living in harmony with nature and

Self-Acceptance

each other while naked and unashamed. In my opinion, it is fair to say that their *Self-Acceptance* was untainted and undeniably pure, *As It Pleased God*.

Then, one day, all of this changed when Adam took his eyes off of his wife, Eve, as she entertained the Serpent. As a result, the Serpent found an open door and tempted Eve through her unforeseen weakness called ACCEPTANCE. Why would she desire acceptance with Adam in the picture? Unfortunately, as he tended the Garden, Eve had a little too much time on her hands.

It is often said, 'An idle mind is the enemy's playground.' Can our minds literally become a playground? Absolutely. If our thoughts became public knowledge, it would bring the ultimate shame, for real, for real! Instead, God, in His infinite nature, prevents what is going on between our two ears from being exposed until we take action or open our mouths.

What about our body language; is that not public knowledge as well? Our body language can give clues, but it does not speak with total accuracy. Here is why: It is through the MIND that we can connect *Spirit to Spirit* with our Heavenly Father. So, it is forbidden territory unless we grant access through our actions, words, or agreements. For this reason, regardless of what or whose playground we are playing on when we are bored, we must become cautious about our words, thoughts, actions, and agreements.

Unbeknown to most, idleness, greed, and boredom are the leading causes of idolatry. Now, my question is, 'Was Eve idolizing God, herself, her husband, his Purpose, the Garden, or the Serpent?' 'Was Eve being greedy?' 'Was Eve bored out of her mind?' No one knows besides God and Eve herself. All I know is that she wanted more! More of what she already had and more of what was FORBIDDEN! Let us continue...

Yes, Eve was a little naive, but it was also Adam's responsibility to keep her hands busy, doing the Will of God

Self-Acceptance

or keeping her joined in on their Divine Purpose. In my opinion, while Adam was out NURTURING and TILLING the Garden, Eve was out twiddling her thumbs with itching ears, which means that she desired more communication. Was the lack of communication Adam and Eve's downfall? Is the lack of communication still our downfall? Was communication that important in the Garden of Eden?

As a result of a communication deficit, the Serpent tempted Eve to eat from the Tree of Knowledge of Good and Evil. From my perspective, she secretly desired to be in Purpose on purpose, similar to Adam.

Am I pulling for straws here? Absolutely not. If the desires were not there, she would have NEVER offered the Forbidden Fruit to her husband. She should have communicated with him first before entertaining strangers with more than a proper greeting. In my opinion, she would have protected him at all costs, even amid her mistakes. But yet, the only communication she had with her husband was tempting him in the same way that the Serpent tempted her.

In her quest for more acceptance, she involved her husband in attaining the Knowledge of Good and Evil. With this act of disobedience, both Adam and Eve's eyes were opened, marking the inception of shame, cognitive *Self-Awareness*, and the onset of Spiritual Duality (opposing forces or principles).

The moment Adam and Eve disobeyed God, what was previously perfect became imperfect to them. While at the same time, it becomes a catalyst for deeper issues, including fear, blame, guilt, and separation. All of these create barriers and roadblocks within the human psyche of mankind. From back then to this very moment, this is echoing through all of our interactions, unless we reintroduce *Self-Acceptance* back into the equation, *As It Pleases God*.

Self-Acceptance

What does reintroducing *Self-Acceptance* mean for us, especially when we already accept ourselves for who we are? In all simplicity, in a world where Spiritual Duality coexists within the Spiritual Realm and individuals, we must get rid of the fear, blame, guilt, shame, and separation from within ourselves first. Once done, we must activate the Law of Reciprocity and spread acceptance outwardly through the use of the Fruits of the Spirit.

Why use the Fruits of the Spirit? First, they were introduced in the Garden of Eden with Adam and Eve, and this is our second chance to get it right Mentally, Physically, Emotionally, Spiritually, and Financially. Secondly, this whole debacle began with love, food, and purpose, and it is going to begin again through us with love, food, and purpose as well. Blasphemy, right? Wrong. Regardless of how we rationalize and justify our issues, problems, or deficits, the biggest issues known to mankind surround the lack of love, food controversies, and the misunderstanding of Divine Purpose (our reason for being). So, let us go deeper...

In cultivating a healthy relationship with food, we also must take into account the relationship we have with the Mind, Body, Soul, and Spirit. Most often, when dieting, we only focus on the physicalities, glorifying slim figures and perfectly toned bodies, without taking into account the innermost being who is crying out or is being silenced. While this is happening, we begin equating weight loss with our self-worth. Although some may not have this issue, some do, and those are the ones *The Bootylicious Body* is targeting.

When dealing with *Self-Acceptance*, it is not just about liking your body; it is also about liking yourself in whatever state you are in. As a matter of fact, it is the key to real health, happiness, and wealth from the inside out, *As It Pleases God*.

What if we are still having health issues, we are not happy, and we are not wealthy, and still accept ourselves for who we

Self-Acceptance

are? If this is the case, there should be a level of peace and joy from within that confounds human reasoning. If not, true self-acceptance is a fleeting statement.

In the Eye of God, the importance of contentment, regardless of the circumstances, will always be on the table, varying between the Mind, Body, Soul, and Spirit. For example, someone may not have a weight problem, but their emotions are all over the place, or they are dealing with mental trauma.

We are all weighted down in some areas that may not be as obvious as being overweight, but the load still must be carried Mentally, Physically, Emotionally, Spiritually, or Financially. For this reason, Paul says in Philippians 4:11-12: *"Not that I speak in regard to need, for I have learned in whatever state I am, to be content: I know how to be abased, and I know how to abound. Everywhere and in all things I have learned both to be full and to be hungry, both to abound and to suffer need."*

In light of the societal standards and Divine Authenticity, as a *Bootylicious Queen*, we cover all of our bases across the board with fundamental and Spiritual Truths.

At the core, to succeed on any level, our perspectives must change, shifting from restrictions to empowerment and from empowerment to lasting transformation and freedom of choice. How can we choose without restrictions? It is hidden in the power of our words. For example, instead of saying, 'I cannot have that,' consider reframing it to:

- ☐ 'I choose not to have that right now.'
- ☐ 'I will have it on my free day.'
- ☐ 'I am opting to make a better choice.'

Self-Acceptance

Does this really make a difference? Absolutely. The positive subtle change in our language, tone, or inflection encourages the psyche in ways that Science has yet to unveil in totality.

For example, it is not wise to correct or yell at a child in a mean, condescending manner. If we do, they will become immune to this behavior, only to emulate it with other children. Well, the psyche is the same way...actually, it is still the same little child hidden within our adult bodies. Meanwhile, if we mistreat or ignore the psyche, it will rebel against us, even if we do not understand what it is doing and why.

Are we considered little children in adult bodies? Yes. In the Bible, we are referred to as Children of God, regardless of our age, status, fame, or fortune. So, the articulation of words makes a difference, even when sternness is required. Proverbs 18:21 clearly tells us: *"Death and life are in the power of the tongue, And those who love it will eat its fruit."*

Over a period of time, rotten words produce rotten fruits. Is this Biblical? I would have it no other way; *"A wholesome tongue is a tree of life, but perverseness in it breaks the spirit."* Proverbs 15:4. Conversely, positive words bring forth positive fruits. Here is what Proverbs 16:24 shares with us: *"Pleasant words are like a honeycomb, Sweetness to the soul and health to the bones."* To sum it all up, according to the Heavenly of Heavens, it is wise to adopt a positive and encouraging inner dialogue to ensure our small victories are won daily with healthy eating habits for long-term success.

The Opportunity

Amid the *Bootylicious Journey* of self-improvement and self-discovery, we need insight...that is, Divine Insight, to be exact. Self-belief, self-trust, and self-understanding provide *The*

Self-Acceptance

Opportunity for us to become better, stronger, and wiser, *As It Pleases God*. Yes, we are taught to trust God, have faith in Him, and understand His Divine Ways. However, we are not often taught to truly believe in ourselves, trust our instincts, master our senses, and understand the Spiritual Compass that lies within. In the Eye of God, all of these attributes underscore the immense power in participating and shaping our outcomes while confronting our doubts, challenges, weaknesses, and idiosyncrasies.

Do we really possess power? Absolutely. We simply need to know it beyond a shadow of a doubt and own it, *As It Pleases God*. 2 Timothy 1:7 says: *"For God has not given us a spirit of fear, but of power and of love and of a sound mind."* So then, where is the power? The power and opportunities are hidden within each one of us based on our commitments.

What do our commitments have to do with anything? We all have commitments to something or someone. In contrast, with the *Bootylicious Body*, we need the right commitments to run our own race, capitalizing on the challenges and opportunities for Spiritual Growth, *As It Pleases God*. Here is what 1 Corinthians 9:24-27 advises: *"Do you not know that those who run in a race all run, but one receives the prize? Run in such a way that you may obtain it."* Moreover, this mindset helps to make the weak strong, the strong humble, and the humble effective.

In a society that often measures success by external accomplishments, wealth, status, fame, fortune, and titles, one of the worst feelings to experience is to win in the eyes of men and feel like a loser from within. What is even worse is when we experience the symptoms of a bona fide loser behind closed doors with our family members because we do not match the image portrayed.

Self-Acceptance

Can this feeling really engulf us as Believers? It happens to us all, especially when God is not in the equation of what we are doing, saying, becoming, establishing, or conveying. More importantly, if we are engaging in the things He hates, then negative feelings will come with the territory, even if we pretend to have it going on. Unfortunately, this is how we find ourselves in a realm of pretense, putting on all types of masks and grappling with self-doubt, over-the-edge anxiety, bad habits, and a sense of unfulfillment.

In the Eye of God, we should never allow the appearance of anyone to deceive us, including ourselves. It is the character traits and heart posture that determine the 'yea or nay' in or out of the Kingdom of God. Thus, *Self-Acceptance* is crucial, especially when life is lifing, and the Vicissitudes and Seasons of Life are doing their job. If we do not accept ourselves, be it good, bad, or indifferent, we will become prone to people-pleasing or seeking validation.

In the relentless pursuit of perfection, if we do not take *The Opportunity* to become a work-in-progress, we may find ourselves between a rock and a hard place. Why would this occur, especially when putting in the work? It is not humanly possible to achieve perfection without God Almighty, being out of Divine Purpose, or not knowing our reason for being. As a result, the longing within the psyche will remain, nudging us away from worldliness to Godliness. We can debate this issue all we like, but it does not change the fact that we are Spiritual Beings having a human experience. Thus, failures and setbacks will occur from the least to the greatest as training and preparation for our next.

Henry Ford once said, *"If you think you can or think you can't, you will always be right."* He also said, *"Failure is only the opportunity to begin again more intelligently."* If you do not examine the reason

Self-Acceptance

behind your WHY, you may miss out on valuable information needed in dropping the weight for your body type or frame.

Eating for emotional gratification and eating to live are two different things. Nevertheless, you must become happy with who you are in the skin you are in to become truly accountable for your successes and failures in life, as well as with your weight.

As a *Bootylicious Queen*, I understand that it is a good feeling for someone to notice and compliment your weight loss efforts. On the other hand, if you are insecure, it will cause you to downplay your weight loss or give up when no one notices or compliments you. Ultimately, it is for this reason that you must lose weight for yourself and your well-being!

In the *Bootylicious Dietal System*, you must set and achieve your goals while tracking your progress without seeking validation from external sources. In addition, to fill the void from within that we all have, you must also equip yourself for all the challenges or emotional woes you may endure by being kind to yourself during setbacks. Unbeknown to most, the positive and negative interplay between your beliefs, thoughts, motivation, focus, and the understanding of your WHY creates powerful emotional intelligence, strategically molding the framework for change and creating win-wins.

In exploring the deeper reasonings for mastering *Bootyliciousness*, the best way I have found to balance the emotional aspects of the *Bootylicious Journey* is to exercise and celebrate small victories. In Earthen Vessels, this is the SECRET to balancing the emotional challenges you will experience from within. Although most people do not tell you to exercise and celebrate to balance yourself Mentally, Physically, Emotionally, and Spiritually, I will!

Most people stop at the physical benefits of exercise, but forgo the other vital aspects that are needed to become truly

Self-Acceptance

successful on this *Bootylicious Journey*. The bottom line is that accountability is your key to success, and it is also the window that will never close on you. As a matter of fact, it is *The Opportunity* for you to become responsible for yourself!

In bridging the gap between where you are and where you are going on your *Bootylicious Journey*, there are many pills, powders, and potions to lose weight. However, you may receive temporary results, especially if you do not learn how to eat properly. Once you stop using them, the weight comes back to ruin your self-esteem, with or without your permission. Thus, you cannot lay the blame elsewhere.

Weight loss products are contingent upon you doing your part in what you are putting into your body, as well as how much you move around. I am not going to say pills, powders, and potions do not work because they very well may. Here is what I want you to understand: Supplements are used to help with your weight loss efforts. It is not designed to be a substitute for discipline and responsibility. A lackadaisical attitude toward weight loss opens the door to pill-popping, as opposed to using diet pills as a TOOL or *The Opportunity* to help you develop a healthy lifestyle.

For the record, there is no magic pill that will healthily melt your weight off; it takes work. It simply gives you enough time to learn how to eat properly and move your body. If you do not learn how to eat, the pounds will come back, and they will come back with a vengeance, bringing back more pounds than you lost. Sadly, this is the double-edged sword of using weight loss products to replace your willingness to take care of your body.

With all hands on deck, the *Bootylicious Body* products work with eating right and moving your body with a Spiritual Approach, period. Our line of products is crafted to work synergistically with your healthy lifestyle choices. Each item

Self-Acceptance

is infused with ingredients designed to nourish not just your body, but also your Spirit, *As It Pleases God*.

The Bootylicious Body: As It Pleases God® is the answer to your prayers. My best recommendation is to discuss your *Bootylicious Journey* with your doctor before beginning the *Bootylicious Dietal Plan*. While doing so, here are a few questions to ask yourself, but not limited to such:

- ☐ What specific health goals am I trying to achieve with dietary supplements?
- ☐ Am I currently getting adequate nutrients from my diet?
- ☐ Have I consulted with a healthcare professional about taking supplements?
- ☐ What type of dietary supplements am I considering, and what are their benefits?
- ☐ Are there potential side effects or interactions with any medications I am currently taking?
- ☐ What is the recommended daily dosage for the supplements I am interested in?
- ☐ How will I monitor and evaluate the effects of the supplements on my health?
- ☐ Am I aware of any potential nutrient deficiencies based on my diet or lifestyle?
- ☐ What quality and safety standards do the supplements I am considering meet?
- ☐ Is the brand reputable and transparent about its sourcing and manufacturing processes?
- ☐ Do I have any allergies or sensitivities that could be affected by these supplements?
- ☐ What are the long-term effects of taking these dietary supplements?

Self-Acceptance

- Am I prepared to commit to a consistent supplementation routine?
- How do these supplements fit into my overall health and wellness plan?
- Could I achieve my health goals through dietary changes instead of supplements?
- What other lifestyle factors (exercise, sleep, stress management) should I consider alongside supplementation?
- Are there any scientific studies supporting the effectiveness of the supplements I'm considering?
- Am I aware of any potential conflicts in my diet that may reduce the effectiveness of the supplements?
- What is my budget, and how will I afford these supplements over time?
- How will I feel if I do not see any results from taking these supplements?

In the *Bootylicious Body* transparency policy, these questions can help guide your decision-making process. Plus, they are designed to ensure that any supplements you consider taking are beneficial and appropriate for your needs. More importantly, the questions serve as a guiding framework, encouraging you to assess your needs thoughtfully and responsibly while becoming a good steward, *As It Pleases God*.

In the real world, please remember, when in *Purpose on purpose*, a well-informed consumer is indeed a powerful one.

In Purpose on Purpose

Amid the self-stewardship of this matter, being a *Bootylicious Queen* is not just about appearance alone. According to the

Self-Acceptance

Heavenly of Heavens, it is about a MINDSET. Unbeknown to most, the mind sends signals to our bodies, indicating that we are in a safe space, thus reducing stress levels. On the other hand, it also sends signals that we are unsafe as well, thus increasing stress levels. Therefore, when dealing with our *Dietal System* on any level, we must become conscious of our thoughts, emotions, words, desires, and triggers.

What does the mindset have to do with our *Dietal System*, our *Bootyliciousness*, or being *In Purpose on Purpose*? Without knowing the reason for our being, there is a longing from within. So, here is what we must know about how the mindset can work in our favor. First, our *Dietal System* is a mindset predicated on how you feel within your own skin while preparing to be *In Purpose on Purpose*. Secondly, being *In Purpose on Purpose* incorporates a mindset of selflessness, self-confidence, self-love, self-care, and self-empowerment, *As It Pleases God* with outright humility. Thirdly, being *In Purpose on Purpose* takes strength and tenacity, especially when helping the next man in the Spirit of Lovingkindness with gleaned knowledge, wisdom, understanding, and know-how.

What does Divine Purpose have to do with anything? When we are out of Divine Purpose or the Will of God, our bodies will react accordingly, even if we do not understand what is taking place. All the psyche knows is that something is missing, and it will sometimes overcompensate in other areas, such as materialism, gold-digging, portraying a certain image, obsession with titles, status, fame, and so on. Conversely, if we embark upon our Divine Purpose, all of this will fade away, allowing us to evolve into our authentic selves.

As a form of empowerment and to find pleasure in the process of your *Bootylicious Journey*, you should incorporate a few things into your daily walk, but not limited to such:

Self-Acceptance

- ☐ Use the Fruits of the Spirit consistently.
- ☐ Behave Christlike.
- ☐ Pray and GIVE THANKS in all things.
- ☐ Meditate and relax the Mind, Body, and Soul.
- ☐ Engage in deep breathing exercises.
- ☐ Repent and become a better person daily.
- ☐ Forgive yourself and others.
- ☐ Nourish the body.
- ☐ Fast on occasion.
- ☐ Laugh and enjoy life.
- ☐ *Make Fitness Fun.*

Can this list really help with purposefulness? Yes, it can. Normal purpose is often described as what drives individuals to pursue goals, cultivate relationships, and strive for personal growth. Our Divine Purpose, on the other hand, is the reason for one's existence, according to our Predestined Blueprint. In addition, it is the key to unlocking our Divine Authenticity from the Heavenly of Heavens.

Our purpose, passion, talents, or Divine Purpose could be the same or totally different based on what God is using to train, nudge, or correct us, or what we do in exchange for the Higher Calling of Christ Jesus. Hypothetically speaking, due to the influence of our parents' aspirations or societal expectations, we pursue a prestigious law degree, only to feel a deeper yearning for a vocation in the medical field as a doctor.

As the whispers of our Divine Purpose grow more deafening, the tugging from within becomes undeniable. Once we come to the crossroads between personal ambition and our Divine Calling with an unmistakable nudge from the Heavenly of Heavens, we must make a decision. Based on the

Self-Acceptance

scenario from above, in surrendering to the Will of God, we become a doctor, *As It Pleases Him*. And, being that we are already a lawyer, He allows us to do both simultaneously in the Spirit of Duality.

How does the Spirit of Duality work from an occupational change? Just because a change is made does not negate the tools, skills, and knowledge gained from the lawyer-to-doctor transition. Here is how it works: First, we have the intellect and persuasive skills of legal counsel as a lawyer. Secondly, with the healing ingenuity, emotional skills, and ethics of a doctor, to save lives while providing wise counsel to healthcare professionals. Thirdly, we have the backing of the Kingdom for being *In Purpose on Purpose*.

Most often, we think the Spirit of Duality applies to good and evil, right and wrong, just and unjust, and so on. Fortunately, it also applies to our wants, needs, and desires, as well as our Dual Purposes, Talents, and Gifts. In bridging gaps in our lives with the tapestry of experiences, it is only wise to add God into the equation of all things, even when we do not understand what is going on or why. Rest assured, when we give it to God, *As It Pleases Him*, He will work that thing...whatever it is or is not out.

My *Bootylicious Queen*, by giving God what He wants, *As It Pleases Him*, He allows us to use the tools we already have, making us better, stronger, useful, and wiser for the Kingdom while turning us into an ultimate POWERHOUSE with a strategic edge. Just know that Divine Purpose supersedes our self-made purposes, reasonings, passions, and desires for personal satisfaction or instant gratification. Above all, know this: Surrendering to the Will of God does not mean relinquishing our dreams, desires, or goals but rather embracing the understanding of our reasons for being,

Self-Acceptance

removing selfishness, ungratefulness, and pompousness from the equation.

Why does Divine Purpose come before all else? It is connected to our sense of being, designed to guide and protect us for its use for a Greater Good. If omitted or overlooked, feelings of aimlessness, dissatisfaction, ungratefulness, and unease will come forth, even if we think we have it going on and are the best thing since sliced bread. One thing is for sure: We will lack peace, harmony, and fulfillment.

Our Divine Purpose acts as a Spiritual Compass, illuminating our Spiritual Journey. It also provides us with Supernatural Direction and Assistance to align our actions, thoughts, and choices amidst the chaos and confusion of everyday life. Cultivating a sense of openness, obedience, and awareness to become a work-in-progress for the Kingdom of God gives us the upper hand in being placed on the leading edge of Divine Wisdom and Spiritual Revelation.

As a *Bootylicious Queen*, when seeking to be *In Purpose on Purpose*, we may not know how Divine Purpose will unveil itself in our lives. Still, we must remain open and receptive to God's Divine Ingenuity, do what needs to be done, learn what must be learned, understand what needs to be understood, heal what needs healing, and overcome what is in our power to do so.

The common denominator in our Divine Purpose is to uplift, inspire, multiply, or bring healing and restoration to others. When we align our self-made purposes with our Divine Purpose, *As It Pleases God*, this is often where the Supernatural happens. How so? When God is in the equation of all things, the obstacles we encounter may serve as opportunities for growth rather than roadblocks, especially when using the Fruits of the Spirit and the Law of Reciprocity. In a Spiritual Flow as such, this is also where seemingly lose-loses become win-wins for the Kingdom of God.

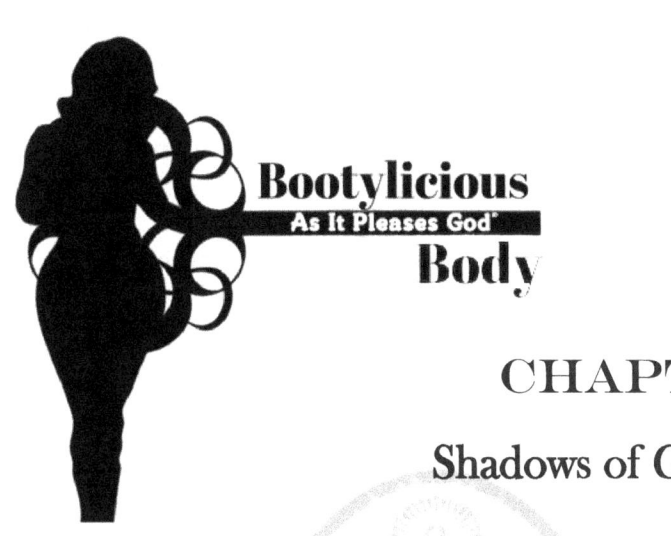

CHAPTER 6

Shadows of Greatness

In the *Shadows of Greatness* and our *Bootyliciousness* will always lie our offspring, be it biological, adopted, or mentored. As we celebrate our achievements, we must also recognize the role we play in the next generation of torchbearers, especially when it comes to the Mental, Physical, Emotional, Spiritual, and Financial Well-Being of the ones we proclaim to love.

In living by example according to our DNA and charactorial traits, the weight of expectations trickles down from us to our children. In the Pursuit of Greatness, if we are not careful about the ideals of success and achievement we portray, we can get a rude awakening by the shadows that become dark and gloomy, drowning out the light, or putting out our spotlight.

Can we control the Shadows of Greatness? Absolutely. Divine Greatness lies within our charactorial development and emotional intelligence, predicated on the use of the Fruits of the Spirit. Outside of the use of the Fruits of the Spirit,

Shadows of Greatness

Divine Greatness is limited. Although we can appear great in our own eyes, it still cannot equate to Divine Greatness or the *Shadows of Greatness* created using the Fruits of the Spirit. Why are they not the same? Greatness in the Eye of God requires positive ambition and nurturing. While, on the other hand, mediocrity requires nothing of us, only to take on a life of its own, as we want life to pander to us through our selfish needs, desires, and habits.

There are Spiritual Laws associated with everything under the sun, except for the use of the Fruits of the Spirit that we learned about in *Temple Maintenance* in Chapter 4. The moment we think we are above reproach or the Spiritual Laws set forth by God, we will get a rude awakening with the Cycles or Vicissitudes of Life.

Unbeknown to most, when life views us as a canker sore, it will arrange situations and circumstances to provoke self-correction. If we avoid corrective or training measures, life will thrust us into a cycle of déjà vu. Is this Biblical? Absolutely. John 15:2 says, *"Every branch in Me that does not bear fruit He takes away; and every branch that bears fruit He prunes, that it may bear more fruit."* Then, Hebrews 12:11 goes on to say, *"Now no chastening seems to be joyful for the present, but painful; nevertheless, afterward it yields the peaceable fruit of righteousness to those who have been trained by it."*

What if we opt out of the pruning and training process? We have free will to opt out, but it does not make us exempt from them. In the reality of our experiences amid opting out, we must understand that Spiritual Duality will still exist, especially in the *Shadows of Greatness*. For instance, based on the Divine Nature of pruning and training, and our freewill options, we will begin choosing disobedience over obedience, unrighteousness over righteousness, selfishness over selflessness, corruption over honesty, unhealthy habits over healthy ones, and the list goes on with the character traits that would bankrupt our nation with strong-armed bullies, using God as a cover-up.

In the *Shadows of Greatness* and *As It Pleases God*, He does not endorse bullies, period! How do I know? Proverbs 16:29 clearly says, "*A violent man entices his neighbor, and leads him in a way that is not good.*" In addition, Proverbs 22:22-23 also says, "*Do not rob the poor because he is poor, and do not oppress the afflicted at the gate; For the Lord will plead their cause, and plunder the soul of those who plunder them.*" As a *Bootylicious Queen*, do not, and I mean do not, engage in bullying others or seek revenge.

Why should we not bully or avenge, especially when it is justified? Unbeknown to most, it places a piercing and targeted bullseye on our health and well-being, especially when children are involved. When living in the Shadows of Greatness, I hold Romans 12:19 close to my heart for Divine Justice: "*Beloved, do not avenge yourselves, but rather give place to wrath; for it is written, 'Vengeance is Mine, I will repay,' says the Lord.*"

The Bullying of Children

In the Eye of God, the adult or child bullies are not the ideal candidates for the *Shadow of Greatness* unless change occurs, *As It Pleases God*. What is the purpose of exempting them? According to the Divine Grace from the Heavenly of Heavens, the exemption is for their PROTECTION. Proverbs 3:11-12 says, "*My son, do not despise the chastening of the Lord, nor detest His correction; for whom the Lord loves He corrects, just as a father the son in whom he delights.*"

From a Divine Perspective, secret or open earthly bullies become Spiritual Bullies once they gain a little power, prestige, or money. Thus, if our charactorial traits are not up to par while operating in Spiritual Disobedience, then it is not wise to play in God's face as if He cannot see us.

What is the big deal about this bullying hoopla? It is difficult to live in a world where children are being bullied because they look different or they are a little chunky. The overbearing responsibility to deal with emotional abuse due to being overweight is overwhelming. It is also challenging for those who become emotional eaters in order to deal with their daily emotional traumas.

How do we recognize bullies? First, the recognition may vary from person to person, trauma to trauma, situation to situation, culture to culture, and so on. Secondly, there are three types of bullies we deal with in this book:

1. Bullying ourselves (Self-Bullying).
2. Bullying others (Traditional Bullying).
3. Bullying God (Spiritual Abuse).

Unbeknown to most, self-inflicted harm is at the top of the list of bullying. Here is why: Without introducing the Spirit of Bullying to ourselves first, we cannot get to the bullying of others or God. In addition, the negative self-talk or thinking is what feeds the Spirit of Bullying that causes a Berating Spirit to manifest. Once we permit it, it will take on a life of its own, with an internal dialogue leading to low self-esteem, anxiety, and depression.

The moment self-criticism, perfectionism, or unrealistic comparisons enter our domain, it is only wise business in the Eye of God to cancel, reject, or reverse them with positivity, scriptures, or affirmations with self-compassion, self-kindness, and self-forgiveness. If not, it will manifest into jealousy, envy, pride, greed, coveting, or self-destruction with a bodacious cover-up, masking the enemy from within.

Shadows of Greatness

To escape from the mindset of inadequacy or negativity, we must identify the character traits of bullying to combat its effect. Nevertheless, for the sake of our *Bootylicious Bodies*, here are a few indicating traits of a bully, but not limited to such:

- ☐ Aggressiveness: Bullies often display hostile behaviors towards others to intimidate, harm, or belittle another person. Unfortunately, relational aggression is the most common downfall of bullies who cross the line with physical abuse, such as hitting, pushing, or any form of physical intimidation.

- ☐ Manipulativeness: Bullies frequently use manipulation to control or intimidate their victims.

- ☐ Lack of Empathy: Bullies typically struggle to understand or care about the feelings of others.

- ☐ Confidence: Bullies may exhibit a strong sense of self-assurance and entitlement that can come off as a lack of humility.

- ☐ Desire Power: Bullies often feel a need to assert dominance over others or pretend as if they are better than someone.

- ☐ Low Self-Esteem: Bullies hide their insecurities behind aggressive or abusive words and behaviors.

- ☐ Thrive on Attention: Bullies often seek out attention, even if it is negative, debauched, or unfavorable.

Shadows of Greatness

- ☐ Social Isolation: Bullies may isolate their victims to exert control over something or someone.

- ☐ Intimidation Tactics: Bullies use threats or fear to manipulate their targets into conforming or obeying.

- ☐ Group Dynamics: Bullies may operate within packs or groups to amplify their intimidation tactics and allegiance.

- ☐ Recurrent Justification: Bullies often rationalize and justify their actions, downplay the impact on victims, or blame others for their behaviors.

- ☐ Hostility Towards Rules: Bullies may show a disregard for rules, regulations, or authoritative figures.

- ☐ Prone to Outbursts: Bullies have sudden displays of anger when challenged or temper tantrums when they do not get what they want. Frankly, this often spills over into verbal abuse that encompasses name-calling, insults, and threats.

- ☐ Project Suffering: Bullies may derive pleasure from the suffering of others, especially if they are of zero benefit to them or their agenda. Moreover, they tend not to care about the consequences until after the fact, or they get caught red-handed.

- ☐ Habitual Behavior: Bullying behaviors a filled with bad and unproductive habits, interactions, or addictions.

- ☐ Projection: Bullies gain their superficial strength by projecting their own insecurities onto others.

Shadows of Greatness

- Social Skills Deficits: Bullies often lack the necessary skills to build healthy relationships with emotional intelligence.

- Denial of Responsibility: Bullies often deny responsibility for their irresponsibility while actively pointing the finger at others.

- Cyberbullying: Bullies use the internet to express their frustrations and aggressions with those in a public setting with the intent to humiliate or bring shame to someone. In addition, it can also be used as a weapon of guilt, imposing harsh judgment, or a tool of disgrace used to spread rumors and destroy lives.

- Rotten Fruits: Bullies usually leave behind a slew of rotten fruits and wounded victims.

Most often, bullies do not realize they are bullies because they are busy trying to protect themselves from predators or wolves in sheep's clothing. Still, these negative behaviors reveal deeper psychological, social, or emotional issues. The more these issues remain unaddressed, they will continue to prevent us from working on ourselves as we should.

In the *Shadows of Greatness*, we must create a safe space for ourselves and others to ensure that the Spirit of God can remain, *As It Pleases Him*. The moment we negate dwelling in safety, the distractions, challenges, and conflicting ideologies may consume us with the Spirit of Confusion, overshadowing the importance of nurturing the psyche.

Shadows of Greatness

When dealing with the psyche of mankind as a *Bootylicious Queen*, we need a few things, but not limited to such:

- ☐ We need love.
- ☐ We need communication.
- ☐ We need diversity.
- ☐ We need inclusion.
- ☐ We need understanding.
- ☐ We need value.
- ☐ We need Divine Communion (Prayer, Repentance, Meditation, Forgiveness, and Worship).

For all of my *Bootylicious Queens*: These things cost us nothing to exhibit, but we can lose everything for not exhibiting them. To avoid the *Emotional Scars of a Child* in an adult body, we must put in the work because most of our adulthood issues or traumas are a result of some form of unresolved childhood scar.

Emotional Scars of a Child

How do we make the *Emotional Scars of a Child* make sense? Picturesquely, when our children cannot run, jump, and play with other children due to rejection, it creates an emotional scar that may affect them for the rest of their lives, primarily if they suppress their emotions through eating. Moreover, it can also affect their individuality and creativity, preventing them from stepping out of the shadows and embracing their true selves. Nonetheless, what we do not realize is that this child never leaves us...even as an adult, this child will remain within the psyche with these same scars unless they willfully heal them.

Shadows of Greatness

Most often, we think that children who are obese cannot run, jump, and play because their bodies will not allow them. But this is so far from the truth; children will play regardless of their size. Whereas, they will refuse to run, jump, and play when they are being mocked, picked on, laughed at, or bullied. This is indeed what damages a child's self-esteem, which causes them to turn to food for comfort.

As a common practice, children should be taught to eat healthily, but this is not always the case because children are fed by their parents. They may have little control over planning their meals or their normal body weight for their age bracket. If a growing child is constantly called fat or told to stop eating, it creates hidden fears and insecurities that may last a lifetime. The fear of eating does not come about when we become adults; it is an underlying emotional or mental trauma stemming from childhood.

As life would have it, we do not talk about children being traumatized by this weight loss craze. In a world that increasingly celebrates conformity, we are raising children to think more about losing weight than living a fulfilled lifestyle. Even when we go to the doctor, they focus on weight loss for our health, but yet pump us full of pills with side effects that decline our health! We have an epidemic here.

Our children are our future; we must understand that eating is normal for children and emotional traumatization is not. They mimic what they see, and if you want your children to become healthy, you must lead by example. Children are conditioned by their environment; if they see bad eating habits, then they will not understand how to do otherwise until they become older and more mature.

In order to safeguard the health of your child or children, you must educate them on eating healthy when they are young to prevent the atrocities of life as much as possible. Allowing our children to overindulge in processed foods can put our children at risk of disease! Take the time to read the label of what you are feeding your children, and I promise that you will think twice about what you allow them to consume. Listen, there are a lot of fake, plastic, and concrete foods that we are feeding our children that are damaging their little digestive tracts. Children are getting bigger for a reason, and it is your responsibility to understand why!

It is best to introduce your children to healthy alternatives by eliminating junk food from your pantry. In addition, you can pack their lunches for school to ensure that you know what they are eating. Fresh fruits, vegetable cups, vegetable or fruit-based snacks, nuts, and frozen yogurts are good, healthy snacks for your children. Get them hooked on drinking water as opposed to juice, and get them active...kids love to play.

Now, if your kids must have some sort of juice, then make it yourself. You can blend fresh fruits and water with a little honey; it makes a great healthy alternative for kids who do not like water. Furthermore, if they are addicted to television or games, it is time to get them actively involved in things that require movement. Trust me, when their bodies are moving, they will naturally crave water!

Children will become more confident when they are busy doing something as opposed to sitting around watching TV, gaming, Instagramming, or Facebooking. Get them into dancing, playing sports, doing chores, etc.; besides, this burns more calories to bring about restoration and renewal within the depths of their soul, keeping the emotional overeating at bay.

Childhood obesity rates are alarming. How do I know? I was one of them. The Bible says that, "*My people perish for the lack of knowledge.*" Processed, fake, and fast foods are taking over. Our children are suffering...we are supposed to keep our children safe. But how can we keep them safe when we are not safe ourselves?

The little that we understand about how food is being processed is detrimental to the health of our children. What do we do? The goal is to keep our foods as close to their natural state as possible, make sure we are eating clean, balanced meals, make sure that our children are pooping properly, get our children more involved in activities, and educate them about how to make the proper choices about diet, nutrition, fitness, and overall health.

No Bounds

When it comes to the *Bootylicious Body*, Divine Greatness knows *No Bounds*, especially when we properly educate ourselves, our children, and others on becoming and remaining healthy Mentally, Physically, Emotionally, Spiritually, and Financially. Although this may be an understatement for some; nevertheless, a Spiritual Approach to education and awareness empowers us, the future, and our next. Thus, we should never allow something or someone to overshadow the Divine Elements of True Greatness, *As It Pleases God*.

Although we are all different, we still should have open discussions, role models, support, and access to viable resources to facilitate the complexities of the human experience with essential and sound Spiritual Principles. After all, the profound and transcendent qualities attributed to the essence of our being already possess everything it needs to grow great, and all we need to do is provide the right conditions for it to come forth with unlimited potential, *As It Pleases God*.

Shadows of Greatness

What does unlimited potential mean for Believers? The *Shadows of Greatness* are already locked up within our loins...all we need to do is use the Heavenly Keys provided as a GIFT to mankind to gain Divine Access. To truly harness the benefits, forming a *Spirit to Spirit* Connection with our Heavenly Father helps to facilitate this process in Earthen Vessels.

In recognizing and accepting this Divine Assistance, *As It Pleases God*, it is imperative to work on our character traits to ensure they become Christlike. If not, we will become Spiritually Blocked to avoid the misuse of our Spiritual Gifts.

How do we work on our charactorial behaviors, *As It Pleases God*? The Spiritual Cheatsheet is wrapped in using the Fruits of the Spirit. Once we perfect them as a *Bootylicious Queen*, it is a wrap! God will move Heaven and Earth with Divine Favor for those who become a work-in-progress using the Fruits of the Spirit consistently in the Spirit of Excellence. By embracing this perspective, we do not need to be perfect...just willing and usable, and all else will take care of itself while helping us to self-correct at the drop of a dime.

For the purpose of the *Bootylicious Body*, we must become aware of three components of releasing our unlimited potential into the Earth. We need:

1. Divine Omnipotence.
2. Divine Omniscience.
3. Divine Omnipresence.

The Divine Omnipotence (All-Encompassing Power) from the Heavenly of Heavens is here to assist us with unlimited power. All we need is faith and hope in Divine Assistance from the Holy Spirit while developing good character traits, *As It Pleases God*. Whether we are on the *Bootylicious Dietal Plan* or living real life with God's Divine Omnipotency, we must confidently know and acknowledge that we are reinforced and maintained by the Holy Trinity, which is greater than ourselves.

Divine Omniscience is available to give us the knowledge and Infinite Awareness (Foresight) needed to move forward in the Spirit of Excellence. For those who are not in the know, the Divine Omnipresence (The All-Knowing God) is with us, transcending physical boundaries to provide unity and the interconnectedness we need among the brethren to feed His sheep.

As God governs all things, including us, with wisdom and love, knowing all things, we cannot hide anything from Him. The moment we think we have one up on Him, we will suffer some form of breakdown Mentally, Physically, Emotionally, Spiritually, or Financially. To be clear, I do not wish a breakdown upon anyone—I am only the Divine Messenger, helping you to help yourself.

Concerning human free will, the goal is to pay attention to what is taking place within your psyche to understand your next move better. It also helps us determine the scripture that needs applying, what must be reversed or counteracted, the forgiveness or repentance that needs to occur, or what we must seek the Lord regarding.

For all of the *Bootylicious Queens*, the Divine Secret to getting in the *No Bounds* Zone, *As It Pleases God*, is to get into His Divine Presence, *Spirit to Spirit*. Then repent, forgive, usher in the Holy Spirit, cover yourself with the Blood of Jesus, give thanks, ask the question, and document the answer. Then, rinse and repeat with the next question.

What if God does not answer? It is okay. As long as the question is documented in your Spiritual Journal, you can revisit it later. Then again, when you least expect it, the answer will come to you. The goal is to become consistent, and the more you exercise your Spiritual Muscle in this area, the stronger you will become and the more He will trust you with Divine Downloads. Until then, just give thanks for the Divine Information in advance and release it.

As a Word to the Wise, sometimes, silence is the answer. God does not like repeating Himself, especially when we have failed to document or we have allowed ourselves to become distracted by the frivolities or pleasures of life. When we attempt to make Him fit into our narratives, we will get the ultimate silent treatment. So, do not take it personally, nor should we become weary or disappointed when this happens. Above all, God is Divinely Omnipresent (Everywhere at Once), so silence should never equate to absence.

In the Eye of God, silence can be a powerful teacher, primarily if used as a moment of introspection and self-reflection. Here is how: Simply document what you are feeling and why you are feeling that way, where it occurred, and with whom. Then align it with the Word of God, doing your part while giving thanks for the lesson or experience. How do I know? I write from experience...the same way that I do what I do, *As It Pleases God*, you can do likewise if you follow instructions.

The Bootylicious Body: As It Pleases God® is designed to get your wheels turning in the right direction to ensure you are not left behind licking your wounds of insecurity. Listen, the *Shadows of Greatness* are at your beck and call. Will you pick up or hang up?

If you allow yourself to feel, to question, and to grow on this *Bootylicious Journey* of faith, *The Commitment* needed, *As It Pleases God*, is all on you. Let us talk about it in the next chapter as you begin to trust the greater tapestry of life.

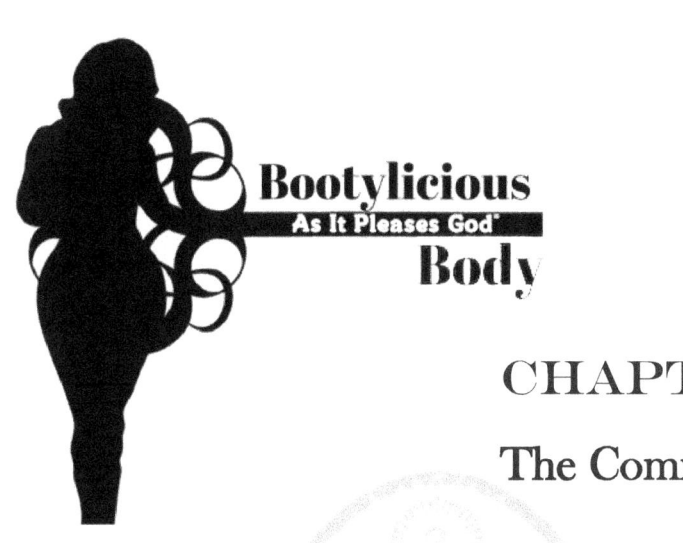

CHAPTER 7
The Commitment

In *The Commitment* to yourself in *The Bootylicious Body: As It Pleases God*®, you must know your why. On the other hand, when it comes to dieting, as a *Bootylicious Queen*, you need to know the REASON behind your why! Is there a difference? Absolutely. One makes a statement, and the other gives the details. In the Kingdom of God, we need both to ensure there is a Spiritual Seal placed on our Earthen Vessels, *As It Pleases God*.

Why must we know the reason behind the why? God is interested in the details, and if we fail to present them when petitioning, then we can limit ourselves, especially when dealing with the NEXT STEP of anything or with anyone.

In *The Commitment*, amid our free will, we also have the option of adding God into the equation of the why and our next steps. Here is how I do it: I would say, *"Speak Lord, your servant is listening."* Or, *"Thank you Lord, your servant hears You."* I gleaned this from 1 Samuel 3:10, and I will allow you to be the

The Commitment

judge of whether I am listening and hearing correctly about our *Bootyliciousness*.

As a matter of fact, when it comes down to your *Bootylicious Queenship*, there is no 'Just Because.' There must be a true understanding of what you are doing and the reason why. It is the clueless dieting that has stolen your power or your self-esteem, and this is your moment to reclaim your rights to a healthy Mind, Body, Soul, and Spirit.

When you find what works for you, you are better able to stick with it. Or, better yet, you are better equipped to 'Do You' with no regrets! Of course, the goal is to lose weight healthily, but what is your reason? In order to find or keep your inspiration, it must run deep...you have to pull that real reason from the depths of your soul. You must be able to look in the mirror without feeling disgusted or guilty. However, it cannot be the only reason why you need to lose weight.

In *The Commitment* process as a *Bootylicious Queen*, we must begin with a Divine Commitment to our Heavenly Father, giving up or placing limits on anything or anyone not conducive to the Will of God in our lives. Once established, we must become a work-in-progress by answering a few questions:

- ☐ What are you committed to?
- ☐ Who are you committed to?
- ☐ Why are you committed?
- ☐ When did you become committed?
- ☐ How did you commit?
- ☐ Where did you commit?
- ☐ What is your vision for the commitment?
- ☐ Where does God fit into this equational commitment?
- ☐ What are your excuses?
- ☐ Do you have any unresolved conflicts?
- ☐ Are you self-disciplined?

The Commitment

- ☐ Are you willing to take a risk?
- ☐ Why do I want to achieve this?

What is the purpose of asking these questions? In a society that demands our right-now attention, querying ourselves helps to pinpoint the reason behind our level of commitment. Using questions as a tool of self-reflection, we can dig a little deeper into our motives to determine our heart and mind postures. Without knowing and understanding the 'Why' behind a commitment, we can lose focus, passion, or desire quickly, squashing our sense of fulfillment.

Most often, we associate commitment with a relationship with someone, but it can also apply to a commitment to something, an idea, a process, or even a system. For example:

- ☐ Personal fitness goals.
- ☐ Education or skill development.
- ☐ Professional projects or deadlines.
- ☐ Family commitments.
- ☐ Volunteer work or community service.
- ☐ Financial savings goals.
- ☐ Health and wellness routines.
- ☐ Social gatherings, parties, or events.
- ☐ Hobbies and creative pursuits.
- ☐ Travel or vacation plans.
- ☐ Home improvement projects.
- ☐ Self-care routines.
- ☐ Reading or learning new things.
- ☐ Attending workshops or seminars.
- ☐ Dietary changes or meal planning.
- ☐ Mentoring or coaching others.
- ☐ Maintaining work-life balance.

The Commitment

Finding the reasons behind your why is not just about pulling reasons out of you; it is about me sharing my reasons as well. As a Kingdomly Servant Lover of other *Bootylicious Queens* like myself, I desire to live as long as possible with good health, wealth, and success to assist them on their unique *Bootylicious Journeys*. In clearing the path for them, they can do likewise for the up-and-coming *Bootylicious Queens* who are in their nesting phases.

The *Bootylicious Legacy* is here to stay forever to empower other *Bootylicious Queens* to own their beauty. Plus, this book is not about being thin; it is about being HEALTHY, FIT, AND FABULOUS!

In between losing pounds, in *The Commitment* Process as a *Bootylicious Queen*, you must build other areas of your life as well, especially your inner health. Most often, when we talk about inner issues, most people are in denial or playing pretend. They will never admit the battles raging from within. Sadly, some people prefer to die with their lies, but for a *Bootylicious Queen* like yourself, this is not an option, right?

Emphasizing self-acceptance and celebrating authenticity, *As It Pleases God*, we must break the negative, unfruitful, and unproductive cycle to prevent self-sabotage. By no means should a *Bootylicious Queen* leave all types of rotten fruits all over the place with no remorse or turn against herself.

What if a *Bootylicious Queen* is clueless about her rotten fruits? First, it is time to get in the know about them. Secondly, following Proverbs 3:5-6 is mandatory: *"Trust in the LORD with all your heart, and lean not on your own understanding; in all your ways acknowledge Him, and He shall direct your paths."*

With *The Commitment* to yourself, Mental, Physical, Emotional, and Spiritual Healing will help to shed the baggage that keeps you holding on to hurt, revenge, defeat, or anger.

The Commitment

My *Bootylicious Queen*, when you treat your body like a Temple, it brings about healing, restoration, energy, and power. Still, amid all, it cannot be about superficial vanity whatsoever.

Overcoming Vanity

As a *Bootylicious Queen*, this cannot be about vanity because it is through vanity that our insecurities are born, bred, and fed. In addition, with this superficial trait, focusing solely on the polished exteriors of individuals unveils the hidden elements of jealousy, envy, competition, hatred, and strife. Rest assured, beneath this surface lies a complex interplay of negative emotions, traumas, and motivations that will become dominant players, shaping our interactions, heart postures, mindsets, and personal narratives. For this reason, Ecclesiastes 1:2 says, " *'Vanity of vanities,' says the Preacher; 'Vanity of vanities, all is vanity.'* "

Why is *Overcoming Vanity* so important when participating in *The Bootylicious Body: As It Pleases God*®? Unfortunately, vainness leads to all types of plotting, schemes, and sabotage due to underlying rage and fear. Even Psalm 2:1 has a question: *"Why do the nations rage, and the people plot a vain thing?"* Thus, when dealing with the *Bootylicious Dietary Plan*, we do not want any negative traits or hormones to hinder our progress, health, or healing process.

As a *Bootylicious Queen*, in accordance with your free will, you must ensure you do not fall in the 'all category' in the '*All is Vanity*' charactorial traits. Listed below are a few ways to *Overcome Vanity*, but not limited to such:

- ☐ Practice Humility: In *Overcoming Vanity*, it is wise to embrace the idea that everyone has strengths and weaknesses while becoming a work-in-progress daily. Recognizing that no one is flawless definitely relieves the pressure of pretense, opening the door to introspection and understanding from a Divine Perspective. In addition, practicing humility helps you to develop and maintain a growth mindset, allowing you to overcome your self-induced stumbling or roadblocks. 1 Corinthians 10:24 says, *"Let no one seek his own, but each one the other's well-being."*

☐ Practice Acknowledgment: To *Overcoming Vanity* in a world that often prizes perfection over reality, it can become extremely challenging to embrace your flaws and imperfections for what they are. Conversely, as a catalyst for growth and self-improvement according to your Divine Design, acknowledging and examining your imperfections will help you work on whatever you have the courage to face. In the Eye of God, you cannot go wrong with owning your truth, bearing your own load while wholeheartedly working on yourself, *As It Pleases Him*. With this approach, it leads to meaningful change and resilience. Galatians 6:4-5 says, *"But let each one examine his own work, and then he will have rejoicing in himself alone, and not in another. For each one shall bear his own load."*

☐ Be Grateful: In *Overcoming Vanity*, becoming grateful for what you have or do not have is one way into the Heart of God. By far, it opens the floodgates to more. In my opinion, gratefulness builds resilience faster than anything when dealing with humility. Without gratefulness, true humility cannot occur, even if we pretend to be humble. In the end, it only makes others

The Commitment

feel undervalued, misused, disrespected, or abused. By far, a mask of humility is very corrosive, and ungratefulness will rat out this charactorial trait faster than anything I know to this date.

Romans 1:21 even says: *"Because, although they knew God, they did not glorify Him as God, nor were thankful, but became futile in their thoughts, and their foolish hearts were darkened."* All in all, the Divine Interplay between gratefulness and humility can work in your favor if you use it, *As It Pleases God.*

- ☐ Seek Constructive Criticism: When *Overcoming Vanity*, we cannot take a backseat on authentic feedback. Surround yourself with honest friends who will tell you the truth or give you helpful feedback with a fresh perspective. When doing so, please keep an open mind while accepting and learning from their insights. While at the same time using it as a tool of growth to become better, stronger, and wiser, rather than getting defensive, negative, or combative.

  In all things lies a nugget of wisdom, and it is our responsibility as *Bootylicious Queens* to glean it, transforming our weaknesses into strengths and a lose-lose into a win-win. Here is what James 1:2-4 says, *"My brethren, count it all joy when you fall into various trials, knowing that the testing of your faith produces patience. But let patience have its perfect work, that you may be perfect and complete, lacking nothing."*

- ☐ Selflessly Focus on Others: When *Overcoming Vanity*, shift your attention from yourself to those around you and become a servant to help others. Philippians 2:3-4

The Commitment

says, "*Let nothing be done through selfish ambition or conceit, but in lowliness of mind let each esteem others better than himself. Let each of you look out not only for his own interests, but also for the interests of others.*" Volunteer, greet people, ask about others' lives, and practice active listening. 1 Peter 4:10 says, "*As each one has received a gift, minister it to one another, as good stewards of the manifold grace of God.*"

- ☐ Limit Social Media Usage: In *Overcoming Vanity*, we must reduce the time spent on negative platforms that promote comparison, ungratefulness, and vanity. Curate your feeds to include positive influences. 1 Corinthians 15:33 says, "*Do not be deceived: 'Evil company corrupts good habits.'*" Protecting the eye gates, ear gates, and the gate of our mouths is of great importance. So, it behooves you to choose wisely, knowing this: "*As iron sharpens iron, so a man sharpens the countenance of his friend.*" Proverbs 27:17. If it is not sharpening you...back up! Although you may get cut from time to time by sharpening influences; yet, you will still heal only to heal another, such as the Cycle of Life.

- ☐ Engage in Self-Reflection: In *Overcoming Vanity*, regularly assess your thoughts, words, desires, and actions. Journaling can help clarify your heart posture, mindset, desires, and motivations. It can also help you identify moments of vanity. Why must we self-reflect? Matthew 15:19 advises: "*For out of the heart proceed evil thoughts, murders, adulteries, fornications, thefts, false witness, blasphemies.*" The moment you think you are exempt from these negative charactorial traits, it means you are smack dab in the middle of them. For this reason, you must actively use the Fruits of the Spirit faithfully and

The Commitment

behave Christlike. If not, you can 'get got' by the enemy's wiles when you least expect it.

- ☐ Celebrate Others' Success: In *Overcoming Vanity*, instead of feeling jealous, envious, or competitive, genuinely congratulate and support others in their achievements. Why should we celebrate others? It helps to prevent instability from within or being two-faced. James 1:8 says, *"He is a double-minded man, unstable in all his ways."*

- ☐ Set Meaningful Goals: In *Overcoming Vanity*, pursue goals that contribute to personal growth or the well-being of others instead of superficial achievements. In whatever you do, follow Proverbs 16:3: *"Commit your works to the Lord, and your thoughts will be established."*

- ☐ Practice Kindness: In *Overcoming Vanity*, acts of kindness can help you develop empathy and compassion, reducing selfishness and self-centeredness. Philippians 2:3 says, *"Let nothing be done through selfish ambition or conceit, but in lowliness of mind let each esteem others better than himself."*

- ☐ Learn from Failure: In *Overcoming Vanity*, embrace setbacks as opportunities to learn, grow, and sow back into the Kingdom while creating a win-win out of everything and with everyone. Here is what Isaiah 41:10 tells us: *"Fear not, for I am with you; be not dismayed, for I am your God. I will strengthen you, yes, I will help you; I will uphold you with My righteous right hand."*

The Commitment

- ☐ Limit Comparisons: In *Overcoming Vanity*, recognize that everyone's journey is uniquely different. Focus on your own path or your Predestined Blueprint while staying in your own lane rather than comparing yourself with others. 2 Corinthians 10:12 says, *"For we dare not classify or compare ourselves with those who commend themselves. But they, measuring themselves by themselves, and comparing themselves among themselves, are not wise."*

- ☐ Challenge or cancel Negative Thoughts: In *Overcoming Vanity*, when you notice negative thoughts, counteract them with positive affirmations that emphasize authenticity over appearance. Can we really cancel or challenge negativity? Absolutely. 2 Corinthians 10:5 says, *"Casting down arguments and every high thing that exalts itself against the knowledge of God, bringing every thought into captivity to the obedience of Christ."*

    If you desire to gain control over the bombarding negativity, you must master dualism, the equal and opposite of everything, willfully interjecting positivity. By far, when doing so, your inner chatter or self-talk will change for the better, guaranteed. As a Word to the Wise, you should never leave negativity AS IS. If you do, it will grow with a formidable yoke! Reverse it to positive and keep it moving in the Spirit of Excellence.

- ☐ Limit Materialism: In *Overcoming Vanity*, reevaluate your relationship with things, possessions, and status, getting rid of anything or anyone leading you into idolatry. What causes materialism? 1 John 2:16 says, *"For all that is in the world—the lust of the flesh, the lust of the eyes, and the pride of life—is not of the Father but is of the*

The Commitment

world." The cause will fall under one or more of the three categories. In addition, it can also fall under a subcategory of power, money, sex, status, fame, or likes.

- ☐ Share with Others: In *Overcoming Vanity*, share your knowledge, wisdom, experience, and skills with others. Teaching others can help you appreciate the value of activating the Law of Reciprocity over showcasing yourself to be seen. Acts 20:35 says, *"I have shown you in every way, by laboring like this, that you must support the weak. And remember the words of the Lord Jesus, that He said, 'It is more blessed to give than to receive.'"*

By shifting your focus in *Overcoming Vanity*, from superficial appearances to values and inner qualities containing health, wealth, and good success, *As It Pleases God*, you will find the inspiration needed to succeed at becoming happy. Yes, truly happy with yourself, as well as becoming the best and healthiest version of yourself, with unspeakable joy.

Now, in *The Commitment* to *The Bootylicious Body: As It Pleases God*®, the power of *Understanding Nutrition* is important. Of course, you do not need to know everything, but there are indeed a few things you must know, such as 1 Corinthians 10:31, *"Therefore, whether you eat or drink, or whatever you do, do all to the glory of God."*

Understanding Nutrition

In Understanding Nutrition, let us introduce Genesis 1:29, *"And God said, 'See, I have given you every herb that yields seed which is*

The Commitment

on the face of all the earth, and every tree whose fruit yields seed; to you it shall be for food.' " In Earthen Vessels, we must understand two things:

- ☐ Macronutrients: Carbohydrates, Proteins, and Fats
- ☐ Micronutrients: Vitamins and Minerals

The Macros and Micros of our nutrients are essential in *The Bootyliciousness* from the *Ancient of Days* to this very moment as the building blocks of nutrition. Although it is not spoken about much in these terms, still, as *Bootylicious Queens*, we need to remain in the know, *As It Pleases God*. More importantly, understanding these nutrients can help us make informed choices about our *Bootylicious Dietal Plan* while enhancing our health and well-being, *As It Pleases Him*.

Regardless of whether we are looking to lose weight, build muscle, or maintain a healthy diet, macronutrients are essential nutrients that our bodies require to function properly. In addition, they also provide us with the energy necessary for daily activities. All of which are crucial for maintaining overall health and well-being according to our DNA, which incorporates carbohydrates, proteins, and fats. Balancing carbohydrates, proteins, and fats looks something like this, but is not limited to such:

- ☐ Carbohydrates: 45-65% of total daily consumption.
- ☐ Proteins: 10-35% of total daily consumption.
- ☐ Fats: 20-35% of total daily consumption.

Carbohydrates are the body's main source of energy, crucial for fueling our physical activities and brain functions. They

The Commitment

are composed of sugar molecules and can be classified into three categories: simple carbohydrates (sugars), complex carbohydrates (starches), and fiber.

- ☐ Simple Carbohydrates are found in fruits, dairy products, and sweeteners. These are quickly absorbed by the body and provide immediate energy. However, they all can lead to spikes in blood sugar if consumed in excess.

- ☐ Complex Carbohydrates are found in whole grains, legumes, and starchy vegetables. They provide a more sustained energy release and are often rich in vitamins and minerals.

- ☐ Fiber is not digested by the body. However, it does play a crucial role in digestive health, helping to regulate blood sugar levels and aiding in weight management by promoting satiety.

Proteins are necessary for building and repairing tissues, making enzymes, hormones, and other body chemicals. They are composed of amino acids, some of which are essential and must be obtained from food.

- ☐ Complete Proteins: These contain all the essential amino acids and are typically found in animal products such as meat, eggs, and dairy. Some plant-based sources, like quinoa and soy, also provide complete proteins.

The Commitment

- Incomplete Proteins: Found in most plant foods, these sources lack one or more essential amino acids. However, by combining various plant foods, such as beans and rice, we can achieve a complete amino acid profile.

Fats are essential for hormone production, nutrient absorption, cell structure, energy storage, insulation, and protecting vital organs. All of which play a crucial role in the absorption of fat-soluble vitamins (A, D, E, and K). In understanding fats in simplicity, they are divided into three main types of fats:

- Saturated Fats: These are typically found in animal products and some plant oils (like coconut oil). These should be consumed in moderation because a diet high in saturated fat can increase cholesterol levels, blocking our arteries.

- Unsaturated Fats: These are considered healthier fats and can be further divided into monounsaturated and polyunsaturated fats. They are typically found in avocados, olive oil, nuts, seeds, and fatty fish. According to our Divine Design, they can help reduce inflammation and lower the risk of heart disease as they can help reduce bad cholesterol levels and promote good cholesterol.

- Trans Fats: These transformed fats are artificially created fats found in some processed foods. As a *Bootylicious Queen*, they should be avoided or reserved for your free day. Unfortunately, they can increase

The Commitment

unhealthy cholesterol levels while lowering healthy cholesterol levels.

Micronutrients are organic and inorganic compounds that are required by the body in minimal quantities, hidden in our vitamins and minerals. Above all, micronutrient deficiencies can lead to various health problems. Consider consulting a healthcare professional or a nutritionist for personalized advice, particularly if you suspect deficiencies or have specific health concerns. By prioritizing micronutrients, it establishes the foundation for long-term wellness and success as *Bootylicious Queens*.

In understanding the difference between vitamins and minerals, here are examples:

- Vitamins:
    - Water-soluble vitamins (including Vitamin C and B-complex vitamins) must be consumed regularly as they are not stored in the body.
    - Fat-soluble vitamins (including Vitamins A, D, E, and K) can be stored in body fat and the liver and are absorbed along with dietary fat.

- Minerals:
    - Major minerals (including calcium, potassium, and magnesium) are required in larger amounts.
    - Trace minerals (including iron, zinc, and selenium) are needed in smaller amounts but are equally important.

The Commitment

The bottom line is that in addition to food, as *Bootylicious Queens*, we must take our supplemental vitamins daily. Whether our supplemental vitamins are chosen or another is preferred, take them! Do not depend on food alone to supply all of your vitamin needs. Here are a few examples of vitamin choices for food, but not limited to such:

- ☐ Vitamin A: Carrots, sweet potatoes, spinach.
- ☐ Vitamin C: Citrus fruits, berries, bell peppers.
- ☐ B Vitamins: Whole grains, legumes, eggs.
- ☐ Vitamin D: Fatty fish, fortified dairy products, sunlight exposure.
- ☐ Vitamin E: Nuts, seeds, green leafy vegetables.
- ☐ Vitamin K: Kale, broccoli, Brussels sprouts.

Here is a checklist for Minerals:

- ☐ Calcium: Dairy products, leafy greens, tofu.
- ☐ Iron: Red meat, beans, lentils.
- ☐ Zinc: Shellfish, meat, seeds.
- ☐ Magnesium: Nuts, seeds, whole grains.

Micronutrients are involved in a multitude of bodily functions, including:

- ☐ Metabolism: Many vitamins and minerals help convert food into energy. For instance, B vitamins play a vital role in metabolizing carbohydrates, fats, and proteins.

- ☐ Immune Function: Certain micronutrients, such as Vitamin C and Zinc, are essential for a robust immune response, helping the body fend off infections.

The Commitment

- ☐ Bone Health: Calcium and Vitamin D are crucial for maintaining bone density and strength.

- ☐ Antioxidant Activity: Vitamins A, C, and E, along with minerals like selenium, act as antioxidants, protecting cells from oxidative stress and reducing the risk of chronic diseases.

- ☐ Cognitive Functions: Some vitamins and minerals are linked to cognitive health. For example, Vitamin B12 is known to support brain health and reduce cognitive decline.

In *The Bootylicious Body: As It Pleases God*®, we must eat a variety of foods and focus on eating whole and unprocessed foods while listening to our bodies. Will our bodies speak to us? Absolutely. Listening to our bodies and building an authentic and healthy relationship with ourselves is designed to send us bodily clues. As a result, it will help to improve energy levels, enhance our moods, and lower the risk of chronic diseases.

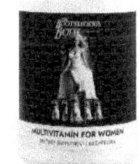

As Dr. Y. Bur, The WHY Doctor, I totally understand that the vitamin talk and hoopla can seem overwhelming at times. To say the least, with an overwhelming amount of choices, it is easy to feel lost amidst the swirling sea of marketing claims and nutritional advice. However, I am here to simplify the process because I believe that achieving your health and wellness goals should be accessible and enjoyable—just like being a *Bootylicious Queen*! As someone who embraces the philosophy of self-love and empowerment, I am excited to share a

The Commitment

carefully curated line of vitamins and supplements. All of which are designed specifically for those looking to enhance their journey toward a healthier, more vibrant life. *The Bootylicious Body* Vitamins and Supplements are aimed at demystifying the complex world of nutrition while bringing you products that support your unique goals and body type.

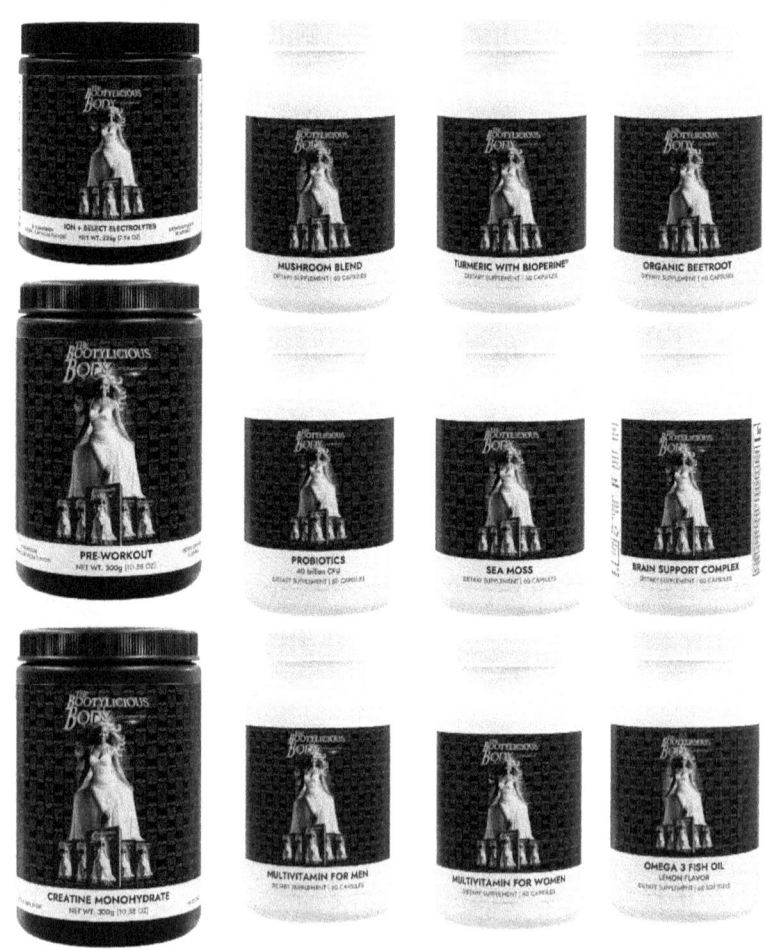

The Bootylicious Vitamins and Supplements
www.BootyliciousBody.com

The Commitment

Embracing your inner *Bootylicious Queen* is not just about looking good; it is about feeling good, empowered, and confident. With *The Bootylicious Body* Vitamins and Supplements, I am committed to turning your confusion into clarity, *As It Pleases God*. Together, let us redefine wellness, one vitamin at a time, as *The Body Speaks in Quinternity* for us, for you, and for them!

The Body Speaks in Quinternity

In the hustle and bustle of daily life, when life is lifing, we often forget to bring our bodies into the equation of what is taking place from within. Our bodies are constantly providing signals that reflect our Mental, Physical, Emotional, and Spiritual states through our senses, conscience, and bodily functions. Often enough, they are presented through fatigue, tension, headaches, discomfort, sleep disruptions, digestive problems, stress, anxiety, or even cravings.

As *Bootylicious Queens*, once we learn to engage with our bodies, we become empowered to live healthier, more fulfilling lives, *As It Pleases God*. Ephesians 5:29-30 says, *"For no one ever hated his own flesh, but nourishes and cherishes it, just as the Lord does the church. For we are members of His body, of His flesh and of His bones."*

How do we get our bodies to speak to us? We must begin asking it questions. Unbeknown to most, the body has a voice, but unfortunately, this is the one voice that is ignored by most. Of course, we pray to God to send us a sign, not realizing the body is one of the best ways in which He communicates with us. Really? Yes, really! The body will tell us everything we need to know if only we listen to it.

The Commitment

The Mind-Body Connection is POWERFUL. How do I know? I use it faithfully, and this is why I share this Divine Information, leading the way, *As It Pleases God*. According to the Heavenly of Heavens, this is not new information. Actually, it is ANCIENT. We have somehow forgotten or lost touch with it until now.

We often look to communicate with God, our Heavenly Father, outside of ourselves. However, in the Eye of God, when communicating, *As It Pleases Him*, we are looking the wrong way. The Divine Communication Tools are already within our bodies; therefore, with *The Commitment*, we need to know this. We do not need to dive into anything spooky or cultic to Divinely Connect to our Heavenly Father, nor should we become brainwashed about Him. Whatever we need to connect to Him, *Spirit to Spirit*, is already within us, ready, willing, and able to assist.

For starters, as *Bootylicious Queens*, here are FIVE things we need to get the ball rolling with the Quinternity of getting the body to speak to us in ways that will trump human reasoning:

- ☐ Willingness.
- ☐ Obedience.
- ☐ Querying.
- ☐ Listening.
- ☐ Documenting.

If we opt out of these five things, the body will withhold information from us, even if we feel entitled. Above all, our Spiritual Discerning faculties will not work as they should, clouding our sense of clarity. As a result, the psyche will begin to speak louder than our Spirit Man, preventing us from waking up from our slumber. Is this real? It is as real as the oxygen we are breathing!

The Commitment

We are a Divine System in the Eye of God; thus, we have the Divine Right to connect to it, *As It Pleases Him*. Now, if we opt out, then we must depend on another man's system to tell us what we should already know, but overlooked. The wealth of information is already hidden within our loins, and it is our responsibility to EXTRACT and CONVERT it.

How do we extract and convert information, especially when we feel clueless? Feeling clueless does not mean that we are. All we need to do is tap into the Divine Reservoir of information by getting *The Body to Speak*. Here are sample questions that I ask most *Bootylicious Queens*, getting their bodies to speak based on their system of conveyance:

- ☐ Are you too busy to cook?
- ☐ Are you too busy to workout?
- ☐ Are you too busy to plan your meals?
- ☐ Are you too busy to take care of your Temple?
- ☐ What is your body saying to you?

These are the questions we need to ask ourselves when we become too busy to help, nurture, and care for our well-being. The hindrance to weight loss has always been hidden in the lack of time. In my opinion, if you take the time to watch the news, watch television, engage in social media, talk on the phone, and so on...you do have time.

From my perspective, the lack of time is an excuse! Here is why I believe what I believe: Matthew 6:22-23 says, *"The lamp of the body is the eye. If therefore your eye is good, your whole body will be full of light. But if your eye is bad, your whole body will be full of darkness. If therefore the light that is in you is darkness, how great is that darkness!"*

The Commitment

The impact of our inner lives really makes a difference in our well-being, determining a guided or misguided vision. With an uplifting perspective, *As It Pleases God*, we will find that *The Body Speaks* to us in ways that will trump human reasoning.

As we strive for this clarity as *Bootylicious Queens*, preparing proper meals and snacks for our dietary needs is essential to our success. When we leave our health up to someone else, we will become disappointed every time. If you have to prepare your meals once a week and then freeze them, please do so. It is no different from eating out. Besides, when eating out, you are not getting freshly prepared food as they would lead you to think. It has been frozen at some point...so do not become deceived by restaurants' shake-and-bake tactics!

As a rule of thumb, in the *Bootylicious Dietary Plan*, avoid buying any PREPACKAGED FROZEN MEALS unless you prepare them yourself. Simply put, you must cook and prepare your own meals. Plus, preparing your meals for yourself and your family in advance puts you in control of your time, and it allows you to become proactive in your meal preparations. Also, keep your freshly cut and cleaned fruits and vegetables readily available to prevent the temptation to snack on unhealthy processed foods.

Five servings a day of fruits and vegetables will help with the desire to snack when you are not hungry. Why five meals? According to the Heavenly of Heavens, we can tap into the Quinternity of our DNA.

The Quinternity is not the same as Quaternity. Here is the deal: Quaternity deals with the Mind, Body, Soul, and Spirit. In contrast, Quinternity deals with the concept or system consisting of five parts or elements. The five essential elements of Quinternity regarding any system are:

☐ Inputs.

The Commitment

- ☐ Processes.
- ☐ Outputs.
- ☐ Feedback.
- ☐ Environment.

In the Eye of God, Quinternity applies to Biological Systems, Business or Operational Systems, Social Sciences or Social Systems, Technology or Automation Systems, and the Body of Christ. In understanding any system for our Heaven on Earth Experiences, whether it be in the context of technology, biology, sociology, or Spirituality, it is crucial to identify and analyze the core components that make it function.

Although not limited, the five functions cater to our bodily systems, human connections, and relationship conduciveness or configuration to create BALANCE. They are connected to the Cornerstone of our thoughts, desires, emotions, words, and actions.

The Geniuses of yesteryear used this Divine Concept and the Power hidden within Quinternity, and so can you. As a *Bootylicious Queen*, you no longer need to wait on trendsetters; you have the power hidden within your loins to become one, *As It Pleases God*.

By paying close attention to the Quinternity associated with elements, individuals, and organizations can optimize varying systems for greater efficiency and effectiveness. All of which have a way of leading to better outcomes and increased adaptability or productivity. Also, when Quinternity is understood, *As It Pleases God*, it helps us blend science, philosophy, and imagination together, opening the four dimensions of Quaternity of the Mind, Body, Soul, and Spirit beyond measure.

The Commitment

How do we make Quinternity make sense? For example, for the Divine System of the hand to work properly in relation to our bodies, we have five fingers on each hand in a normal setting. Then again, we have five toes in a normal setting to support each foot. If we miss one toe or finger, an imbalance will occur. Even if we somehow have an extra finger or toe, an imbalance will still occur as well. Nevertheless, when the body feels balanced, *As It Pleases God*, it will speak louder than it would for those who do not include Him at all.

Listen, when *The Commitment* is in full effect as a *Bootylicious Queen*, the conscience speaks, the senses speak, the psyche speaks, the mind speaks, and most of all, energy speaks to us through our bodily senses, urges, and demeanor. Thus, we must learn how to listen effectively, regardless of whether we are in or out of the Kingdom of God.

We do not need to overcomplicate Quinternity; keep it simple, and it will work as it should. Just use the example of the hand with any system, using a five-finger countdown of what, when, where, how, and why for questioning and imaginative exploration. Does it work? I have a stamp of guarantee on it, especially if documentation occurs, whether or not the Voice of God is speaking.

Why do we need to document information? It opens the Floodgate of Wisdom, Divine Wisdom, to be exact. When God can trust us to become the portal of information to help ourselves and others, He will trust us with more. If we do not document, He will not trust us to become a conduit with the transfer of information.

For instance, when someone attempts to impress me with how much they know about God or convince me of their Divine Eliteness, I take into account what is documented. Here is the deal: Revelation 12:11 says, *"And they overcame him by the blood of the Lamb and by the word of their testimony, and they did not*

The Commitment

love their lives to the death." With the information we are entrusted with, Isaiah 30:8 tells us what to do with it: *"Now go, write it before them on a tablet, and note it on a scroll, that it may be for time to come, forever and ever."*

In addition, the importance of vision, systems, plans, and Testimonies, writing them down and acting upon them with faith and diligence, is required of us. We may not be able to write a book, still, as *Bootylicious Queens*, there is no reason not to take notes. Here is what Habakkuk 2:2-3 says about this matter: *"Then the Lord answered me and said: 'Write the vision and make it plain on tablets, that he may run who reads it. For the vision is yet for an appointed time; but at the end it will speak, and it will not lie. Though it tarries, wait for it; because it will surely come, it will not tarry.'"*

What if we have a photographic memory? Photographic memories do not impress God. Is it not He who gave it? More importantly, if we use our photographic memories for our benefit only, unfortunately, in the Eye of God, it is a misuse of the GIFT. Plus, when we consume our own fruits without sharing, *As It Pleases God*, the body will begin to withhold information from us or do weird stuff as the hole from within becomes a pit.

Our Spiritual Gifts are not for our benefit only; they are designed to feed God's sheep to benefit the Kingdom. Please allow me to Spiritually Align this: 1 Corinthians 12:4-7 says, *"There are diversities of gifts, but the same Spirit. There are differences of ministries, but the same Lord. And there are diversities of activities, but it is the same God who works all in all. But the manifestation of the Spirit is given to each one for the profit of all."* We must leave a trail of information for the next in line, and if we are not doing so, it is time to get busy because the Spirit of Quinternity is role-calling.

The Commitment

In addition, we can also symbolically associate Quinternity with what Believers call a Five-Fold Ministry for equipping the Saints. The Body of a balanced Ministry, according to Ephesians 4:11-13 says, *"And He Himself gave some to be apostles, some prophets, some evangelists, and some pastors and teachers, for the equipping of the saints for the work of the ministry, for the edifying of the body of Christ, till we all come to the unity of the faith and of the knowledge of the Son of God, to a perfect man, to the measure of the stature of the fullness of Christ."*

In *The Commitment* to the *Bootylicious Body*, in the same way that the Body of Christ speaks, with the proper use of Quinternity, *As It Pleases God*, our bodies will begin to tell us things that will trump human reasoning. The state of being in a harmonious relationship with our bodies, ourselves, and our Heavenly Father plays a pivotal role in this *Bootylicious Dietal Journey*.

As It Pleases God, embracing our unique Quinternity of body types, like the celebrated term '*Bootyliciousness*,' allows us to transcend the superficial judgments often imposed by society who do not understand the Divine Framework bestowed. *The Commitment* to our bodies is not merely about physical appearance; it challenges us to cultivate a deep sense of respect and admiration for ourselves, *As It Pleases God*.

According to the Heavenly of Heavens, our physical form is an expression of our Spiritual Essence of our Divine Interconnectedness with a pearl of profound Heavenly Wisdom. All we need to do is tap into it, *As It Pleases God*.

Now that we have gotten *The Commitment* out of the way, let us move on to *The Bootylicious Secrets*.

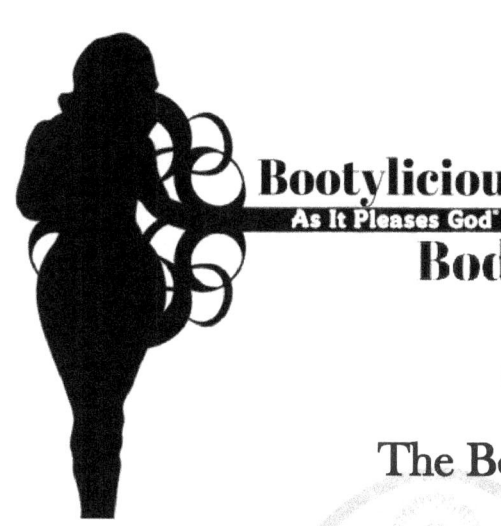

CHAPTER 8

The Bootylicious Secrets

It is often said that a secret is no longer a secret once it is exposed. Nonetheless, based on our perceptions, secrets can do two things: unify or divide. In this chapter, with *The Bootylicious Secrets*, in all transparency, we are going to do both in a good, healthy way. As we delve into the dual nature of secrets, the goal is to overcome these silent barriers, *As It Pleases God*.

When it comes to eating healthy, many of us find ourselves in a whirlwind of choices, often leading to all types of confusion. Nor do we know where to begin. So, we opt for everything that says healthy, low-calorie, diet, low-fat, no-fat, and so on. Not realizing these deceptive terms are the types of processed foods contributing to our weight gain or lack of weight loss. In addition, they often come with loads of hidden sugars, unhealthy fats, and additives that do not benefit our bodies whatsoever. *The Bootylicious Body: As It Pleases God*® does not restrict these products; we limit them and consume them on our free days!

The Bootylicious Secrets

Why are unhealthy items not restricted? First, we operate with Biblical Principles of free will and choices in the *Bootylicious Dietal Plan*. Forced obedience will cause the human psyche to rebel, especially when it is unresolved trauma, causing us to make unwise or unhealthy choices. If God does not force us to do anything, then our *Bootylicious Dietal Plan* will not either.

Secondly, if one has been eating a certain way for 40 years, it is not wise to make them go cold turkey unless it is a willful choice to do so. In this phase, it is only wise to begin to learn more about what is being consumed and why, gaining more knowledge. Why is knowledge so important in the *Bootylicious Dietal Plan*? Once again, we deal with Biblical Principles in the *Bootylicious Dietal Plan*. Here is what Hosea 4:6 says about knowledge: *"My people are destroyed for lack of knowledge. Because you have rejected knowledge, I also will reject you from being priest for Me; because you have forgotten the law of your God, I also will forget your children."* So, to avoid the destruction of generations, we choose to educate the *Bootylicious Queens* instead of forcing them.

Thirdly, we do not force our *Bootylicious Queens* not to have something they like; we simply establish a timeframe. Because Proverbs 4:7 says, *"Wisdom is the principal thing; therefore get wisdom. And in all your getting, get understanding."* Once the timeframes are understood from a Divine Perspective, we can definitely apply wisdom and common sense in our choices while developing self-control, *As It Pleases God*.

Lastly, when we eat clean 80% of the time, our bodies will naturally reject junk, getting rid of it. Here is a secret: Once we begin to feel the difference in how it makes our bodies feel, we will naturally avoid the foods the body rejects. Above all, as a *Bootylicious Queen*, while mastering our food intake, we must also develop our character by monitoring its output.

The Bootylicious Secrets

If we can manage what is going into our bodies without monitoring our heart postures, it means that our issues are running deep in the Eye of God. Here is the Spiritual Alignment punchline according to Matthew 15:17-20. *"Do you not yet understand that whatever enters the mouth goes into the stomach and is eliminated? But those things which proceed out of the mouth come from the heart, and they defile a man. For out of the heart proceed evil thoughts, murders, adulteries, fornications, thefts, false witness, blasphemies. These are the things which defile a man, but to eat with unwashed hands does not defile a man."*

What does defilement have to do with anything? The concept of defilement is often tied to moral judgment and the choices individuals make regarding their bodies and lifestyles. In the Eye of God, it is wise to stop judging people for their free will choices of food, be it healthy or unhealthy. Instead of criticism, we should provide sound information, wiser choices, and healthier options for them to choose from.

As *Bootylicious Queens*, with a profound understanding and respect for all mankind, how we make people feel in the conveyance process matters. Now, before moving to *The Natural Way*, our purity and righteousness are not determined by food; we determine them by our Moral Compass and the CHARACTORIAL FRUITS we bear in or out of season.

The Natural Way

In a world saturated with diet trends, fads, and quick fixes, the pursuit of a healthy lifestyle according to our genetic makeup leads us back to the basics. Whole foods are foods that are minimally processed, close to their natural state, and free from artificial ingredients that retain their essential nutrients, fiber, and flavor. Picturesquely, this includes foods such as fruits, vegetables, whole grains, nuts, seeds, legumes, fish, and lean meats.

As a *Bootylicious Queen*, if you are looking for *The Natural Way* of dieting, emphasizing whole foods rather than processed options, then continue reading. The *Bootylicious Dietal Plan* has a lot of great tips and information to sustain your Mind, Body, Soul, and Spirit, empowering you to evolve into the best version of yourself.

My *Bootylicious Queen*, it is imperative that you cook your own food and move your body frequently to avoid falling into the trap of convenience unless it is your free night. Even though fast food, takeout, and pre-packaged meals seem like the quickest solutions for your lifestyle. But if they cost you your health and well-being, the price is too high. Use them as a reward or celebratory factor and not as a lifestyle. Listed below are a few reasons why a *Bootylicious Queen* should prepare her own meals 80% of the time, but not limited to such:

- ☐ Control Over Ingredients: A *Bootylicious Queen* can prepare meals with fresh, whole ingredients and avoid unhealthy additives, fillers, and preservatives.

- ☐ Portion Management: A *Bootylicious Queen* can serve appropriate portions to help with calorie control and prevent overeating.

- ☐ Cost Efficiency: A *Bootylicious Queen* can save money compared to dining out or ordering takeout, especially when buying in bulk.

The Bootylicious Secrets

- Customization: A *Bootylicious Queen* can tailor meals to match her personal dietary needs and preferences, making healthy eating more enjoyable.

- Nutritional Awareness: A *Bootylicious Queen* can increase awareness of what she is consuming and its nutritional value.

- Meal Prep Convenience: A *Bootylicious Queen* can prepare meals in advance to avoid the temptation of quick, unhealthy options on busy days.

- Boosts Cooking Skills: A *Bootylicious Queen* can develop her cooking skills, leading to greater satisfaction and success in maintaining healthy habits and body type.

- Mindful Eating: A *Bootylicious Queen's* home-cooked meals encourage her to eat more mindfully, slowing down her chewing to savor flavors and textures.

- Healthier Cooking Methods: A *Bootylicious Queen* can choose healthier cooking techniques like steaming, grilling, or baking instead of frying.

- Avoid Tempting Extras: A *Bootylicious Queen* can avoid the extra calories often found in restaurant meals, such as dressings, sauces, condiments, and sides.

- Encourages Variety: A *Bootylicious Queen* can try new recipes and ingredients, promoting a varied and balanced diet.

The Bootylicious Secrets

- ☐ Family Involvement: A *Bootylicious Queen* can create a social environment, involving her family and friends in meal preparation while fostering healthy habits together.

- ☐ Satisfaction and Enjoyment: A *Bootylicious Queen* can create meals that can be fun, enhancing her relationship with food.

- ☐ Reduced Risk of Diet Sabotage: A *Bootylicious Queen* can reduce the hidden calories and unhealthy options that can derail her dietal efforts.

- ☐ Learning and Experimentation: A *Bootylicious Queen* can experiment with ingredients and recipes, making healthy eating more exciting.

- ☐ Understanding Nutrition: A *Bootylicious Queen* can prepare her own meals, increasing her knowledge about the healthiest nutritional choices for her body type.

- ☐ Long-Term Habit Formation: A *Bootylicious Queen* can establish long-lasting, healthy eating habits.

- ☐ Empowerment: A *Bootylicious Queen* can take charge of her life by fostering a sense of accomplishment and ownership of her health journey.

Once a *Bootylicious Queen* takes ownership of her decisions and body, *As It Pleases God*, she is less likely to complain about the small changes leading up to big results.

The Bootylicious Secrets

The Complainers

The biggest complainers are those who do not have anything to do. When you become a couch potato with little or nothing to do, your mind will create things, real or imagined. When the mind is too idle, it creates an imagined hunger in the body! Plus, if you are watching television, the subliminal food messages will become overwhelming because you are allowing the television to dictate your real or imagined urges of hunger.

We can pretend as if we are in control as much as we want, but if the mind is stressed, depressed, or idle, it is easily manipulated if one does not understand what is taking place.

Once again, the *Bootylicious Dietal Plan* is not about vanity, low-fat, or no-fat; it is about making the right choices. When dieting for the wrong reasons or eating the wrong foods, especially when we have unresolved issues or traumas, it can create additional hunger pains. How do I know? By far, hunger is the biggest complaint when dieting; however, you do not want to increase the hunger when you do not have to.

Conversations about body image and eating habits have become increasingly prevalent, especially on social media. For sure, be it secretly or openly, you are not alone in the way you feel about your body or your eating habits. In the United States, we face a myriad of health, well-being, and psychological issues related to weight, from obesity to eating disorders, feelings of inadequacy, frustration with dieting, or guilt over food choices.

According to the Centers for Disease Control and Prevention (CDC), the prevalence of obesity has significantly increased over the past few decades. Unfortunately, this indicates that many individuals are grappling with their relationship with their bodies, a relationship with food, and

The Bootylicious Secrets

other underlying issues, leading to low self-esteem, anxiety, and even depression.

As if that is not enough, we have drug stores on every corner, and they are continuing to grow, outnumbering grocery stores or teaming up with them. It is often said that it is hard to lose weight naturally. My *Bootylicious Queen*, naturally, is by far the best and safest way.

As a rule of thumb, it is important that you do not keep on eating the same foods over and over again, as you will get bored. It does not matter how good they taste; you must get creative in your meal preparations, or you will get tired of eating the same foods. When you cook your food, eat healthily, and exercise...success will come. Remember, Rome was not built overnight; therefore, you must invest in yourself, and your body will invest back into you.

How can our bodies invest in us? Unbeknown to most, our digestive system is often referred to as our second brain. Although most people think that our sexual organ is the second brain, but it is NOT in the Eye of God. Actually, it has its own brainial functions, still it is not a necessity for sustaining life. Therefore, it must take a back seat to our digestive system.

The second brain of our digestive system will tell us what we can or cannot digest. In addition, this hidden and invisible brainial function helps to break down our food, absorb nutrients, and signals us when something is not quite right. It is just a matter of whether we pay attention or listen to the messages our body sends us.

Here is the twist: Suppose we are categorized as one of *The Complainers*. In this case, with the Spirit of Complaint, it will come with blinders or a victim mentality. In so many words, we will most often miss the silent cues of being bloated after a meal, experiencing discomfort after consuming dairy, becoming lethargic after meals, or getting a boost of energy after eating certain items. Then again, as a victim, we may exaggerate our condition to gain sympathy. So, my question is, *'Can You Digest It?'* Why this question? The second brain will respond as long as we place a demand on it, a Spiritual Demand to be exact!

As *Bootylicious Queens*, and *Spirit to Spirit*, we formally place a Spiritual Demand on our digestive system to bring it into Divine Order and Balance, *As It Pleases God*. With this being said, let us go deeper.

Can You Digest It?

The question, 'Can You Digest It?' seems like a no-brainer. Yet and still, the answer to this simple question is loaded with wisdom, Divine Wisdom to be exact.

Digestion begins in the mouth and continues through the stomach and intestines, where the real magic happens. When we consume food out of pleasure, necessity, or convenience, here is how our second brain assesses it: Are the proteins, fats, and carbohydrates suitable or sustainable? Do we have the enzymes necessary to break it down? What vitamins can be extracted or converted? What needs to be rejected? How am I going to make them uncomfortable for their acts of disobedience? How am I going to flush this food out to make room for more?

In essence, our bodies are constantly investing in us, and as *Bootylicious Queens*, we must do our part and identify the negative patterns between certain foods. If not, our bodies will begin to fight back. Really? Yes, really! For example, those who are lactose intolerant may experience gastrointestinal discomfort after consuming dairy products. Due to their body's inability to digest lactose, a sugar found in milk, it fights back the best way it knows how.

The Bootylicious Secrets

As we move on, everyone's digestive system will not process meat correctly. The only way to determine if your digestive tract is resistant to meat products is to remove it temporarily. If you go to the bathroom regularly after removing meat products, then your system is not processing meat properly. If you continue to eat meat, you will eventually end up with some form of colon problem or some form of cancer in your body. When meat sits in your body too long, it rots! When this happens, it overloads your body with unwanted and unneeded toxins that will eventually make you lethargic or sick.

One of the biggest issues faced by *Bootylicious Queens* is the inability to digest beans without the gas and bloating. These small but mighty legumes are packed with nutrients, offering numerous health benefits, including improved digestion, weight management, and heart health.

If you decide to add beans to your diet for protein and fiber, make sure you soak the gases out of your beans first with a tablespoon of baking soda to break down some of the complex carbohydrates responsible for gas. Under no circumstances do you cook dry beans without cleaning and soaking them first to help neutralize the pH and further aid in the breakdown of these troublesome compounds. Here are the steps to soak beans the *Bootylicious* way:

- ☐ Rinse the Beans: Start by rinsing your dried beans thoroughly to remove any dirt or debris.

- ☐ Prepare the Soaking Solution: In a large bowl, combine your rinsed beans with enough water to cover them by a few inches. Add a tablespoon of baking soda to this water.

The Bootylicious Secrets

- ☐ Soak the Beans: Let the beans soak for several hours or, preferably, overnight. During this time, the beans will absorb water, swell, and begin to break down some of the compounds that contribute to gas production.

- ☐ Rinse Again: After soaking, drain and rinse the beans thoroughly under cold water. This step helps to wash away any residual baking soda and the byproducts released during soaking.

- ☐ Cook the Beans: Proceed to cook your beans by boiling or simmering them according to your recipe. Proper cooking ensures that beans are tender and safe to eat.

Adding beans to your diet can lead to numerous health benefits, including increased protein and fiber intake.

The Queen's Secrets and Tips

The use of coconut oil and okra is *The Bootylicious Body's* best-kept secret. When you add these two powerhouse products to your diet, your digestive system will thank you.

Okra is an ancient, super vegetable that is rich in essential nutrients, containing dietary fiber, vitamins such as vitamin A, vitamin C, B6, and vitamin K, and minerals such as magnesium, potassium, and calcium. In addition, it also aids in digestion and helps maintain a healthy gut while facilitating regular bowel movements, preventing unwanted constipation.

Furthermore, okra, also called the Lady's Finger, is extremely low in calories. As a Staple of Greatness, okra has benefits for women that science has yet to discover. However, when cooked, it becomes a little slimy, but we should never allow the slime to fool us. Okra is packed with antioxidants, such as quercetin, catechin, and vitamins C, K, A, B6, and Folate. These compounds help combat oxidative stress in the body, reducing the risk of chronic diseases like heart disease and cancer. While simultaneously helping to stabilize blood sugar levels by slowing down sugar absorption in the intestines and preventing spikes in blood sugar levels.

Okra contains a small amount of healthy fats, specifically omega-3 and omega-6 fatty acids, which can help lower cholesterol levels, especially when paired with fatty fish. For the *Bootylicious Queens*, this is an excellent dish that you will grow to love its benefits, especially when getting creative with okra and fish.

Okra's potassium content also aids in blood pressure regulation, supporting cardiovascular health. So, you see, as a *Bootylicious Queen*, it is beneficial to add okra into our dietal regimen. Here are a few delicious ways to enjoy this nutrient-packed vegetable:

- ☐ Gumbo: A classic dish in Southern cuisine, gumbo features okra as a thickening agent. This savory stew can include various proteins and is perfect for showcasing okra's unique texture.

- ☐ Stir-Fries: Sautéed okra with garlic, onions, and bell peppers makes for a tasty side dish. The quick cooking method retains its nutrients and adds vibrant color to your plate.

- ☐ Okra Chips: For a healthy snack, try baking or air-frying sliced okra until crispy. Season with your favorite spices for a crunchy alternative to traditional chips.

The Bootylicious Secrets

- Soups and Stews: Add okra to soups and stews for added nutrition and thickness. Its unique texture helps enrich the overall dish.

- Salads: Slice fresh okra and toss it into your salads for a vibrant crunch. Its mild flavor works well with dressings and complements a variety of ingredients.

- Smoothies: For a nutritional boost, blend okra into your smoothies. Its mild flavor and thick texture can enhance the drink without overpowering other flavors.

Coconut oil, on the other hand, is rich in medium-chain triglycerides (MCTs), which provide quick energy and can aid in weight management. Coconut oil is considered one of our SUPERFOODS, suitable for frying, sautéing, and baking, and an excellent substitute for butter.

Coconut oil can help improve the absorption of fat-soluble vitamins (A, D, E, and K) and antioxidants, ensuring that your body gets the most out of the foods you eat. The lauric acid in coconut oil has anti-inflammatory properties, which can help in reducing inflammation and promoting overall well-being.

The Bootylicious Body: As It Pleases God® portion secret is based upon the Quinternity System, as spoken about in Chapter 7. As a rule of thumb for a *Bootylicious Queen,* you have five fingers for a reason...you need five servings of fruit per day and five servings of vegetables. Each serving will fit into the palm of your hand, and these servings are MANDATORY! It may seem like a lot, but you will grow accustomed to it. The hand of a *Bootylicious Queen* is her power...therefore, everything she needs is already in her hands!

The Bootylicious Secrets

As we all know, water hydrates the body, and our bodies will actually think it is hungry when it is really thirsty. Therefore, as a Bootylicious *Queen*, before eating, you must consume a warm cup of water, tea, or coffee. Decaffeinated is always best, but with a *Bootylicious Queen*, it is not required unless you have plateaued. If this happens, you must adjust your calorie and clear fluid intake. Also, make sure you are eating your fruits, vegetables, beans, and lean meat while switching up your workout routine to ensure that your body is feeling different movements to other areas of your body.

Green Tea is an Ancient Beverage, standing the test of time. Not only is green tea good for the human body, but it may also proactively lower the risk of neurodegenerative diseases. In all simplicity, it is good for increasing your mental clarity and providing a more stable boost of energy without the jitters. The thermogenic properties of green tea help *Bootylicious Queens* burn calories and increase fat oxidation. All of which are due to a high concentration of catechins, particularly epigallocatechin gallate (EGCG), which have been found to elevate metabolic rates.

Some may disagree, but for a *Bootylicious Queen*, apple cider vinegar is excellent for the body as well. If you can add it to your morning water, that is great. But, if you cannot, make the apple cider vinegar into a warm tea with or without honey. A tablespoon a day of apple cider vinegar is all you need...it increases weight loss, reduces cholesterol, lowers high blood pressure, and helps with arthritis.

When embarking upon this journey, you need to determine if you are going to devote your time to it. If you go into it with a bad attitude, complaining about the food, and hating to move your body, then you may be setting yourself up for defeat. But if you are dedicated to your *Bootylicious Dietal Plan*, success will become your portion! Now, getting down to the

The Bootylicious Secrets

nitty-gritty, there are a few habits that we need to kick in order to succeed in this program:

- ☐ No sodas, not even diet sodas or carbonated drinks, unless it is your free day.
- ☐ Stay hydrated with water, a minimum of 8 cups a day.
- ☐ No artificial flavors.
- ☐ No processed meats, fresh meat only.
- ☐ No packaged meals.
- ☐ Watch out for the hidden sugars.
- ☐ Only eat out of a saucer plate. If this is not possible, eat only half of your meal and save the rest for later.
- ☐ Fresh or frozen fruits or vegetables only, no canned fruits or vegetables.
- ☐ When eating, choose between your meal or dessert. You CANNOT have both in the same meal.
- ☐ Limit television; food commercials will invoke food cravings.

According to the *Bootylicious Dietal Plan*, here is how to take charge of your weight loss in total humility:

- ☐ Overlook the fad diets; they come and go. You are looking for a lifestyle change.
- ☐ Set realistic goals: *The Bootylicious Body* is designed to work with your lifestyle.
- ☐ Make a commitment: Write down some important reasons for changing your eating habits.
- ☐ Start a food diary and record everything you eat. You can also record your emotions as well.
- ☐ Be consistent, and do not give up.

The Bootylicious Secrets

- ☐ Be flexible, even if you make a mistake or eat off plan, then start over the next day with a clean slate.
- ☐ Plan your meals in advance.
- ☐ Congratulate yourself often.

The key to *The Bootylicious Body* is MODERATION. What is moderation? I am so glad you asked! It is the avoidance of excess by exercising self-control; basically, it is eating only what you need to fuel your body without becoming greedy. Our version of moderation is knowing when to eat and what to eat.

Our *Bootylicious Dietal Plan* is not designed to starve you; it is designed to give you freedom with a few restrictions, like eating five to six small meals each day, spaced apart by about three hours within a certain time frame. If gluttony of food is our weakest link, then we need to check and see what is going on within the soulish realm. Why is there an issue? It is all connected! The Mind, Body, Soul, and Spirit should always want the best for you. Now, if the best is not coming forth, there is a blockage somewhere within the psyche, regardless of whether we are small, medium, big, extra large, or anything in between.

It is often said, 'Anything worth having is worth working for.' For me, I will concur, especially when it comes down to your health! Taking one extra step a day toward your goal will get you to your final destination a whole lot faster with the least amount of effort as opposed to not doing anything. It may take a few minutes out of your day to focus on being healthy Mentally, Physically, Emotionally, and Spiritually. But trust me, or even if you do not trust me, time speaks for itself. One minute will eventually add up to 1 whole hour, and one hour will eventually add up to 24 extra hours toward your journey of establishing a balanced and healthy lifestyle.

The Bootylicious Secrets

Once you become cognizant of the value of your time, you are then able to implement or introduce healthier ways of thinking into your daily lifestyle on your own terms or *As It Pleases God*. Once again, it is our MINDSETS that are going to keep us balanced in the way we appropriate the time spent on preparing and maintaining our healthy lifestyle on the go.

In properly governing time, according to the Ancient of Days, the *Bootylicious Dietal Plan* begins with a food diary. Record everything you eat, what you were doing at the time, and how you feel. Doing so tells you about yourself, your temptations, and the emotional state of being that encourages you to eat or snack.

In addition, documenting will indeed pinpoint the emotional triggers preventing you from losing weight or overeating. Do not worry; we all have triggers—some are self-controlled, and some are not. However, you must know what they are to ensure you do not turn on yourself and to become better equipped to deflect or reject the triggers. This strategic approach will help you lose more weight once you see how much you are really eating and why. Here are a few of *The Bootylicious Body* tips:

- ☐ Instead of eating a piece of candy, simply brush your teeth.

- ☐ If you cannot fight off the temptation to cheat or eat badly, allow yourself one bite and throw the rest away. It may seem like a waste of food, but it works!

- ☐ When hunger pains hit you, drink a glass of water, herbal tea, or juice, and wait 10 minutes before eating to see if the hunger passes.

The Bootylicious Secrets

- ☐ Set attainable goals. In the beginning, do not set a goal saying, 'I want to lose 50 pounds.' Make it small, saying, 'I want to lose 5 pounds a month.'

- ☐ Get enough sleep, 7-8 hours is enough.

- ☐ Try to avoid sugar. Sweet foods invoke the craving for more sugary foods.

- ☐ Drink eight glasses of water a day. Your first glass of room-temperature water must be on an empty stomach in the morning. Water is a natural diuretic, and it helps to cut down on your water retention. It will also prevent you from overindulging by causing you to feel full, especially when you squeeze a piece of lemon, lime, or orange into your water. Drinking water also wards off infections and diseases by giving your system an adequate flush.

- ☐ Diet with a friend or join a support group to keep you motivated.

- ☐ Indulge in different activities when the food cravings hit you or when your emotions cause you to want to binge. It is best to go to the gym, take a walk, or indulge in a hobby; it will definitely take your mind off eating.

- ☐ Please do not buy the foods that tempt you; leave them on the shelf at the store. Now, if the desire does not go away, buy and consume it only on your free day. If you have tempting leftovers extending beyond your free day, throw them away! Is this not wasting food?

The Bootylicious Secrets

   Maybe or maybe not; however, it symbolically teaches the mind portion control and rationing.

- [ ] If you have a craving for sugar, grab a piece of fruit such as an orange slice, grapes, berries, etc.

- [ ] You are only allowed one reward night per week or a 24-hour window, such as from Friday at 6 p.m. to Saturday at 6 p.m. This window is the most ideal and the most effective window for *Bootylicious Queens* because it feels like 2-days, but it is technically one. Plus, you can enjoy family time a little better without feeling deprived. In this Bootylicious Dietal Plan, you can use this timeframe as a free day or fasting day, whichever works best for you. Do you!

- [ ] You must weigh yourself once a week at the same time.

- [ ] Use a saucer to eat meals and leave something on your plate. No 'Super-Size' meals, period; if you eat out, a kid's meal is ideal.

- [ ] Do not shop when you are hungry—eat before you go, period.

- [ ] Avoid consuming large quantities of fattening drinks; this includes alcoholic beverages.

- [ ] Keep plenty of foods like raw vegetables and popcorn as snacks between meals.

- [ ] Lose weight only for you.

The Bootylicious Secrets

- ☐ Chew your food nice and slow, savoring every moment!

- ☐ Do not skip meals.

- ☐ Exercise 3-4 times a week, and make sure you stay hydrated.

Your goal is to become healthy, NOT THIN! Your body will find its natural setpoint, and if your setpoint is thick, thin, or anything in between, then so be it!

What is a setpoint? In biological terms, a setpoint often refers to the range in which our body functions optimally regarding weight, temperature, and even mental health. For instance, when we speak about weight setpoints, we recognize that our bodies have a natural range that they tend to maintain, influenced by genetics, metabolism, and lifestyle factors. A setpoint is nothing to be ashamed of, nor should we discredit the setpoint of another. In the union of the Mind, Body, Soul, and Spirit, we not only find health but a deeper connection to ourselves and the way God uniquely created us.

All in all, as *The Bootylicious Secrets* are no longer secret, you must become happy with the frame and *The Divine Canvas* that God has BLESSED you with. And with my PROMISE to you, if you follow instructions, HARMONIOUS JOY will become your portion.

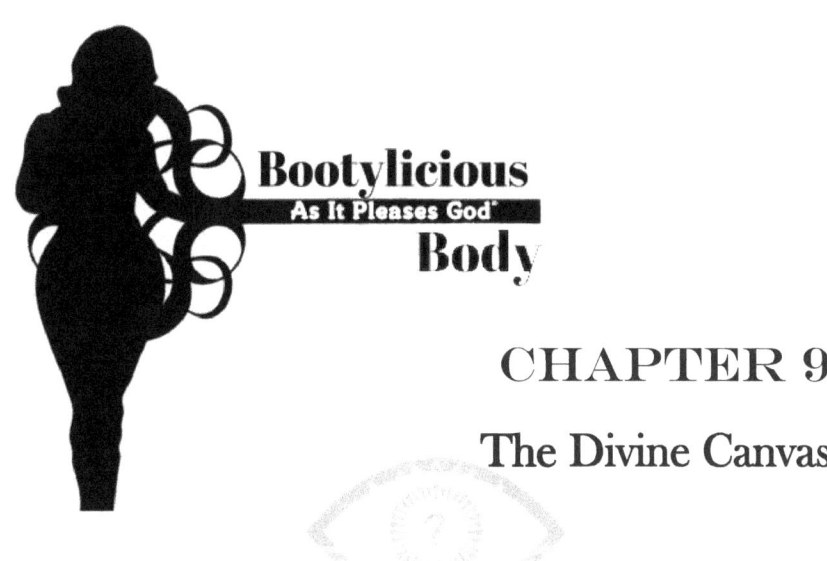

CHAPTER 9
The Divine Canvas

This book, *The Bootylicious Body*, does not want you to feel as if it is a major sacrifice; it is designed to help you develop a healthy, natural lifestyle. Better yet, as real life would have it, it is not about becoming a fitness fanatic; it is about incorporating clean eating and movement into your life. I have found that the most painful part of losing weight is the physical activity aspect. The pain of being sore, the pain of getting tired, and the pain of being bored have plagued us for the longest. Well, this type of mindset stops here!

From my understanding of the *Bootylicious Roots*, we did not have gyms back in the day, we did not have personal trainers, and we did not have liposuction. Yet, the *Bootylicious Queens* were more healthier and fit back then than we are now. So, what is the problem? What do we need to do? We need to get BUSY MOVING IN LIFE. The luxuries of life have caused us to stop moving as much as we should. We are good at counting calories and not our movements...we need to get up with a mission!

When incorporating physical activity, you should mix it up. This ensures that you do not get bored...you can add in your hobbies, walking, cleaning, playing, gardening, etc. The goal is to get creative...calories are calories; it does not matter how you burn them as long as you do. I would suggest that you create fitness opportunities to replace your lengthy workouts. On your break, walk up and down the stairs; when you go to the restroom, do twenty squats; when walking to your car, take the long way or walk around the building first. You will be surprised at the ways you can create hidden opportunities to move your body each day.

Dieting alone is unlikely to bring you the body of your dreams; therefore, you have many options. Yoga, Pilates, cycling, and dancing are the in things right now. If you have gotten off track, renew your commitment to yourself and get moving.

If you are having a hard time losing weight, lacking motivation, or if you are feeling hopeless, get help! Find a support group to help you. If you need a partner to diet or exercise with, then feel free to get one. However, my *Bootylicious Queen*, you do not want to become codependent, nor do you want to become incompatible with those you are partnering with. So, in this chapter, we will learn how to do two things: *Harness Your Power* and *Avoid Judging*. All of which are based on Spiritual Principles designed to make your *Divine Canvas* a masterpiece with zero shame attached.

When your Mind, Body, Soul, and Spirit begin to reflect the true essence of who you are, free of shame and limitations, anchored in love, you are better able to tap into your inner strength without dominating others or being dominated. In *The Divine Canvas*, it is your Divine Authenticity and Uniqueness that assist in removing known and unknown

The Divine Canvas

barriers, helping you come to terms with who you were created to be in Earthen Vessel as a *Bootylicious Queen*. Remember, every stroke on your *Divine Canvas* contributes to the beauty lying within, *Harnessing Your Power* to inspire others to do likewise.

Harness Your Power

As *The Divine Canvas* from the Heavenly of Heavens, regardless of your decisions, you must *Harness Your Power*. It is not conducive or wise to team up with someone who drains you or who is constantly comparing themselves to you. According to Kingdom Standards, this is the ultimate no-no! You will find that a lot of *Bootylicious Queens* roll solo when it comes down to their Mental, Physical, Emotional, and Spiritual Well-Being. Most *Bootylicious Queens* experience better results, success, support, and motivation with classes, personal trainers, or a mate, as opposed to having a buddy system with unlike minds.

The Divine Canvas of a *Bootylicious Queen* knows her worth. And if you desire to become the crème de la crème with Heavenly Poshness, you must know a few things. As fad diets would have it, some people diet to achieve a sexy body, some people diet because they are self-conscious, some people diet because they are ashamed, some people diet to keep up with the Joneses, some people diet for health reasons, and some people diet for a new lifestyle. My *Bootylicious Queen*, once again, you must know the reason behind your why! Remember, you are a tribe of your own. You are the trendsetter, and if you are not setting the right trend with the Divine Greatness that is already within you, you must go back

The Divine Canvas

to the drawing board for self-analysis or self-renewal of your lineage.

My *Bootylicious Queen*, you were born to move...you were born to be active...you were born to be creative...you were born to be healthy. If, for some reason, you are not in that place right now, it is your responsibility to get up, put your crown on, and claim your Throne! Your Spirit Man has been crying out for the truth about the GREATNESS that resides from within.

Based on *The Divine Canvas* set forth, sickness, disease, obesity, and lethargy cannot have us. I invoke the *Spirit of Queenship* right now in the Name of Jesus. The issues of life can no longer weigh our *Bootylicious Queens* down. Our power can no longer be suppressed! Thus, we are taking our bodies back and coming into our own by Divine Decree.

Now, in order to know what works for you as a *Bootylicious Queen* and *The Divine Canvas* set forth, you must follow your instincts first while asking and answering these fact-finding questions:

- ☐ How do you feel about your health?
- ☐ Are you eating properly?
- ☐ Are you receiving the appropriate nutrients daily?
- ☐ Are you on target with your wellness goals?
- ☐ How do you feel about your body?
- ☐ Are you embarrassed about your appearance?
- ☐ Do weight-related issues make you feel awkward?
- ☐ Are you worried about what others are thinking of you?
- ☐ Do you have time to participate in a wellness program?
- ☐ Do you have time to workout?
- ☐ How many times are you able to attend meetings, go to the gym, or attend classes?
- ☐ Does the workout schedule fit into your lifestyle?

The Divine Canvas

- ☐ Are you willing to stick to a weight loss or wellness regimen?
- ☐ How much are you willing to spend on your health and wellness program monthly?
- ☐ Why are you investing in your body?
- ☐ What are your measurements?

Measurements

Right Arm						
Left Arm						
Chest						
Waist						
Hips						
Right Thigh						
Left Thigh						
Weight						
Date						

The truth of the matter is, it does not matter if you are more than 5, 10, 20, 50, or even 100 pounds over your ideal weight; you are at greater risk of potentially deadly conditions, such as diabetes, high blood pressure, heart disease, high cholesterol, and cancer, if you do not eat properly. Not only that, if you are eating processed foods, eating too much meat, or avoiding exercising or moving your body, you are at risk as well. Above all, if you have a health issue, please exercise extreme caution to avoid further damage.

If you have a sedentary lifestyle and are fully able-bodied, it puts you in an extremely high bracket of other health issues and complications. My *Bootylicious Queen*, all you need to do is begin to reprogram your mind.

The Divine Canvas

When you change how you think about yourself, your body will follow. If you think that you are a *Hot Mess*, your body will begin to reflect it. If you think that you are *Sick*, your body will reflect it. If you think that you are *Healthy*, your body will reflect it. When your mind gives up on you, your body will as well. You must master the power of your mind to ensure that it stays powerful, strong, and positive during all phases of life, even if you have Mental, Physical, Emotional, Spiritual, or Financial issues.

When you have a relaxed, focused, and positive state of mind, you will lose more weight, period! The body follows what the mind is feeding it, with or without your permission. My *Bootylicious Queen*, we have a natural desire and instinct to lose weight, improve our appearances, and improve our health as we become older, wiser, and more iconic.

Of course, some people take the easy way out by abusing their bodies with unnecessary surgeries due to hidden insecurities. Although some are needed and are lifesaving for others, you still have the free will to choose, regardless of your reasoning.

Avoid Judging

Amid all this, the act of judging others has become almost second nature. The age-old adage, 'Never judge a book by its cover,' serves as a poignant reminder for myself and others. The tendency to criticize or condemn must be addressed when it comes to *The Divine Canvas* of God. We do not know what He is doing or what He is using to train, test, mold, or position us. Thus, we must exercise extreme caution when judging others because we never know if the judged shoe will be placed on our feet.

For example, life has a way of humbling us, especially when public shaming, private slander, online harassment, and

The Divine Canvas

turning up our noses are involved. Personally, some of the things I judged harshly in one phase of my life are the same things that came back to save my life in another phase. The funny thing about it, I did not remember the underhanded slander and harshness until God brought it to the forefront for repentance and forgiveness. All of which served as a poignant reminder for me, yes, I said me, to always build the esteem of others without destroying them. Primarily, when not having all the facts or using a human perspective, perpetuating a negative cycle without invoking a Divine Perspective or putting things on a positive trajectory, *As It Pleases God*, puts us in the hot seat.

In cultivating a more empathetic view, life has a way of making an example out of us, even the best of us. Mistakes and misjudgments are part of the human experience, allowing us to learn, grow, and sow back into the Kingdom when called upon. Similar to what I am doing now for all of the *Bootylicious Queens*, regardless of age, size, or creed, while choosing my words carefully with no shame attached.

Let me say this before moving on: When dealing with *The Divine Canvas*, we never know when we might find ourselves in a similar situation to what we judged with a rod iron, so a little kindness goes a long way. Here is what Matthew 7:1-2 says, *"Judge not, that you be not judged. For with what judgment you judge, you will be judged; and with the measure you use, it will be measured back to you."*

In a world filled with differing opinions, free will, and varying perspectives, just use the Fruits of the Spirit to examine and behave Christlike to always remain in a zone of safety, allowing Good Measures to become our portion. How is this possible? First, there is no law against the use of the Fruits of the Spirit. Secondly, Luke 6:37-38 says, *"Judge not, and*

The Divine Canvas

you shall not be judged. Condemn not, and you shall not be condemned. Forgive, and you will be forgiven. Give, and it will be given to you: good measure, pressed down, shaken together, and running over will be put into your bosom. For with the same measure that you use, it will be measured back to you."

As *The Divine Canvas* has turned full circle, I have embraced my lessons. I have now become the Teacher, sharing Divine Information for a time such as this.

As a *Bootylicious Queen*, I encourage you to embrace your *Bootyliciousness*. Being overweight is in the eye of the beholder because everyone is not designed to be thin. Thirty-five percent of Americans are unable to prevent being overweight; thus, we must begin to love our genes and the skin we are in.

The *Bootylicious Body* is not a diet of EXCUSES; it is a diet of OWNERSHIP! Yes, owning who you are, owning your body, owning your life, owning your self-perception, owning your vanity, owning your social acceptance, owning your interactions, and owning what you put into your body. Moreover, when taking ownership or authority over the Mind, Body, Soul, and Spirit, *As It Pleases God*, it may sometimes require a fast.

We will discuss the process of fasting in the next chapter to ensure that we all have equal access to *The Bootylicious Freedom* hidden in plain sight.

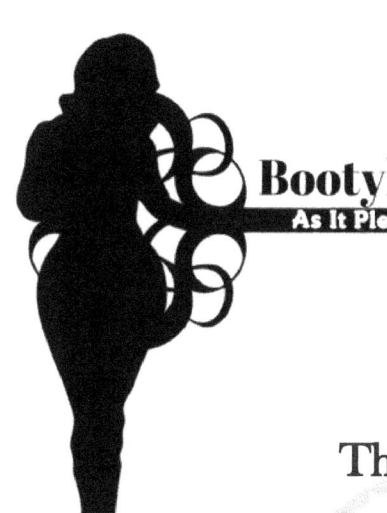

Bootylicious Body — *As It Pleases God*

CHAPTER 10

The Bootylicious Freedom

Everything possessing the Breath of Life has a ticket of Freedom attached to it, called fasting. Fasting is often seen merely as a dietary choice or a Spiritual Practice, but it holds within it the Essence of Freedom, *The Bootylicious Freedom*, to be exact. The concept of fasting transcends just abstaining from food alone. Spiritually Speaking, in Earthen Vessels, fasting symbolizes a deeper liberation that is reflective of our connection with the Cycles of Life, holding profound keys to unlock truths hidden within our existence and DNA.

Regardless of whether we use fasting for purification, reflection, and Spiritual Awakening, it is here to serve us with deeper introspection and reconnection to God, *Spirit to Spirit*. Reclaiming our freedom from societal norms and expectations surrounding food and consumption, as *Bootylicious Queens*, we can chart the heights of Divine Elevation beyond human comprehension.

The Bootylicious Freedom

Now, the moment we begin using the Fruits of the Spirit and behaving Christlike, *As It Pleases God*, it then takes us to another Spiritual Level that most can never attain. Why not? It takes work, and we are held to a higher accountability than most. Luke 12:48 says, *"But he who did not know, yet committed things deserving of stripes, shall be beaten with few. For everyone to whom much is given, from him much will be required; and to whom much has been committed, of him they will ask the more."*

Nevertheless, fasting in the Eye of God is a pathway to *The Bootylicious Freedom*, breaking the chains of all types of bondage, including food. More importantly, it helps to break the little urge from within the psyche to sabotage people, places, and things that we seemingly have the power over, especially when dealing with children, older people with or without disabilities, and people experiencing poverty. For instance, we know beyond a shadow of a doubt that a person is sickly and in need of medical attention. And we, out of spite, attempt to do everything in our power to prevent this person from receiving the life-saving medical treatment or medication needed to survive...God has an ISSUE with this!

What is the purpose of knowing about the urge to sabotage people, places, and things while fasting? We, as Believers, are required to show compassion, and fasting without true compassion to manipulate and control with debaucherous intents or efforts can put a monkey-wrench in our efforts.

Then again, engaging in willful ill will can also create generational curses that our grandmother's washing powder cannot wash off. In addition, it also has a way of placing us or our loved ones in bondage until repentance occurs. Can this really happen to us? It is happening all around us, primarily where envy, jealousy, coveting, greed, competitiveness, and discrimination are occurring, even if it is underlying.

The Bootylicious Freedom

In this day and age, it is disheartening to acknowledge that some individuals are driven by spite to the extent that they would interfere with another person's access to life-saving medical treatment, medication, or safety. From a Spiritual Perspective, interfering with their freedom to live unveils a depth of malice that contains devastating ramifications in the Realm of the Spirit. Here is 1 John 4:20 take on this: *"If someone says, 'I love God,' and hates his brother, he is a liar; for he who does not love his brother whom he has seen, how can he love God whom he has not seen?"*

Actively seeking to undermine another's chance at survival or to prevent someone from having a *Spirit to Spirit* Relationship with our Heavenly Father creates a double-edged sword from the pews to the pulpit and beyond. If one does not believe this, here is what Proverbs 24:17-18 advises: *"Do not rejoice when your enemy falls, and do not let your heart be glad when he stumbles; lest the Lord see it, and it displease Him, and He turn away His anger from him."*

As a *Bootylicious Queen*, this troubling behavior prompts us to explore the intricate relationship between human emotions, particularly spite, and the ethical implications that arise when those emotions lead to harmful actions or decisions against others.

Why is compassion a necessity in the Eye of God? Simply put, compassion is misunderstood by most and used by few, especially when fasting, *As It Pleases God*. Let me explain: Most of us, as Believers, think that compassion is just about sympathetic pity or feelings of empathy. Yet, we miss the fact that it also contains a Spiritual Contingency Clause that is usable and enforceable. What is it? It is associated with the genuine concern for the suffering or misfortunes of others.

The Bootylicious Freedom

"Bear one another's burdens, and so fulfill the law of Christ." Galatians 6:2.

More importantly, if we are the spiteful cause of such suffering or misfortune, we inadvertently ration our own portions. What are our portions? They will vary depending on our heart and mind posture, intent of personal vendetta, or underlying emotions that fuel such decisions. Even Proverbs 14:31 forewarns: *"He who oppresses the poor reproaches his Maker, but he who honors Him has mercy on the needy."* If we unwittingly perpetuate harm due to ingrained biases, we can bring this issue back to our own HOUSE or BLOODLINE. For this reason, it is wise to extend the Spiritual Principles of CARE and COMPASSION to all mankind. Here is what Philippians 2:3-4 says, *"Let nothing be done through selfish ambition or conceit, but in lowliness of mind let each esteem others better than himself. Let each of you look out not only for his own interests, but also for the interests of others."*

Suppose compassion is missing from the equation, *As It Pleases God*, or we allow our personal grievances to overshadow the fundamental human right to health and well-being of His sheep. In this case, real freedom cannot occur. Instead, we must settle for the illusion of freedom while bound, gagged, or blinded by the lust of the eyes, the lust of the flesh, and the pride of life. For my *Bootylicious Queens*, here is the need-to-know from 1 John 3:17-18, *"But whoever has this world's goods, and sees his brother in need, and shuts up his heart from him, how does the love of God abide in him? My little children, let us not love in word or in tongue, but in deed and in truth."*

Why are illusions our only option when having free will? Operating in the Spirit of Spite and jeopardizing human lives for the sake of personal grievances or money grabs places us in a Spiritual Chokehold, publicly or privately. Unfortunately, it zaps freedom from within the human psyche, which allows

The Bootylicious Freedom

the Spirit of Bondage to consume us while the DEMONS from our past, present, and future ride us like a HORSE in the night hours, even if we proclaim Holiness. Is this Biblical? Absolutely, and I would have it no other way, but I must answer this question in two parts.

In the first part, when Job was being challenged, wrestling with questions of suffering and Divine Justice, here are a few questions I want to highlight: *"Have you given the horse strength? Have you clothed his neck with thunder? Can you frighten him like a locust? His majestic snorting strikes terror."* Job 39:19-20. The lies we tell about ourselves and others must stop.

In the same way we fuel the fire in our lives, we can put it out as well. In the Realm of the Spirit, most of our issues are self-induced or self-created by our actions, thoughts, beliefs, words, and character traits. Even if we project, reject, or deflect, it does not negate what is taking place from within.

In the second part, the bottom line is that we need faith to gain freedom over anything or with anyone. If not, Spiritual Epilepsy or Paralysis can consume us or our loved ones. As *Bootylicious Queens*, this is not a Spiritual Taboo; these are Spiritual Facts that we underestimate and overlook, leaving our Bloodline vulnerable. Here is what Matthew 17:14-21 says about this matter: *"And when they had come to the multitude, a man came to Him, kneeling down to Him and saying, 'Lord, have mercy on my son, for he is an epileptic and suffers severely; for he often falls into the fire and often into the water. So I brought him to Your disciples, but they could not cure him.' Then Jesus answered and said, 'O faithless and perverse generation, how long shall I be with you? How long shall I bear with you? Bring him here to Me.' And Jesus rebuked the demon, and it came out of him; and the child was cured from that very hour. Then the disciples came to Jesus privately and said, 'Why could we not cast it out?' So Jesus said to them, 'Because of your unbelief; for assuredly, I say to you, if you have faith as a mustard seed, you will say to this mountain, 'Move from here to there,' and it will move; and nothing will be impossible for you. However, this kind does not go out except by prayer and fasting.'"*

Clearly, I do not wish Spiritual Epilepsy or Paralysis upon anyone, especially innocent bystanders or children. Still, we must know this information as *Bootylicious Queens*, and the only way to break this or clean the Spiritual Slate is to engage in *The Fasting Process* with the *As It Pleases God* approach with love. Above all, fasting or not, to maintain a *Bootylicious Body* from the inside out, remember this: *"Love does no harm to a neighbor; therefore love is the fulfillment of the law."* Romans 13:10.

The Fasting Process

Fasting in the Eye of God develops the discipline of the Mind, Body, Soul, and Spirit. Denying our flesh is becoming more and more a thing of the past, and if we do not refocus, putting our fleshly desires into their proper perspectives, we will self-destruct. Even if we are battling with some sort of health issue, we should not make this an excuse for not fasting. There are so many abridged versions of fasting, appeasing God all the same, regardless of our conditions.

In my opinion, it very well may be a possibility we are sick due to the buildup of toxins in our bodies because we do not fast. However, other forms of fasting provide meaningful benefits; therefore, it is best to check with our Doctors regarding which food fast would best suit our health condition.

The sacrificial need to allow our flesh to hunger, thirst, or desire will bring forth Spiritual Discipline. Why is discipline so important? Our external discipline determines or sets the stage for our internal discipline. For example, if someone proclaims to be a Spiritual Elite, I consider their discipline

The Bootylicious Freedom

from the outside in. I pay attention to their method of operation as it relates to immaterial things, such as:

- ☐ Their level of respect for God, themselves, and others.
- ☐ Their level of proactiveness, filling a need beforehand.
- ☐ Their level of follow-through or follow-up.
- ☐ Their level of helpfulness.
- ☐ Their level of selflessness.
- ☐ How they manage their time.
- ☐ How they manage their emotions.
- ☐ How well they follow instructions.
- ☐ How well they deal with a crisis.
- ☐ How they exhibit self-control under pressure.
- ☐ How they respond to those they do not need.
- ☐ How well they resolve conflict.
- ☐ How well they reverse negatives into positives.
- ☐ How committed they are to their spoken words.
- ☐ How dedicated they are to their God-Given Mission in life.

In the Realm of the Spirit, in or out of our fasting state, our People Skills set precedence over many mind-controlling innuendoes.

The most common innuendo I have heard that we can all relate to is, 'Cleanliness is next to Godliness.' Well, from my perspective, first and foremost, it is not Biblical. Secondly, it is a form of manipulation, dividing us based on appearance. And thirdly, cleanliness or purification scriptures in the Bible refer to cleansing the inside of ourselves via the Mind, Body, and Soul.

Why is inner cleansing so important? From experience, I have met the most organized people, who are nasty and outright evil, squashing anyone who appears beneath them. Yet, they were haunted by their hidden inner demons while

The Bootylicious Freedom

calling me for help as their life continued to spiral downward into the abyss. And, until they changed their perception of life and toward people in general, they could not break the yoke. Why am I telling this story? If we clean the outside, forgetting about cleansing the soul, we can become easily defiled Mentally, Physically, Emotionally, and Spiritually. And, in due time, the joke will be on us.

Just so we are clear, cleanliness is essential for proper hygiene, but when we incorporate God into the equation, we must target the heart first. Why the heart? Because God will send His Chosen Vessels into some really dirty, stinky places to pull out His sheep. If we get into the mindset of turning up our noses at something or someone without lending a helping hand, we have a sincere issue from within in need of reckoning.

What is the big deal? God may require us to get our hands dirty, *As It Pleases Him*. If we are afraid of a bit of dirt, we are not fit for the Kingdom. How is this possible? If we cannot deal with dirt, it is a possibility that we cannot deal with ourselves due to some form of known or unknown identity crisis.

The moment we forget who we are or how we got here, this is the moment the digression process starts to bring us back home to the dirt from the inside out. Really? Yes, really...let us take it to scripture, *"By the sweat of your face you shall eat bread, till you return to the ground, for out of it you were taken; for you are dust, and to dust you shall return."* Genesis 1:27. So, we should never become ungrateful regarding our point of origin or the way God is using the lives of others to accomplish His Divine Purpose, especially if we are not doing our part, we are outright out of purpose, or we do not have a clue about our reason for being.

The Bootylicious Freedom

With all that being said, *The Fasting Process* helps us align ourselves, *Spirit to Spirit*. God has created our bodies in a certain way that complements fasting. On the other hand, if we do not fast, we cause our body to work against itself. For example, when animals get sick, they will instinctually stop eating. Even though they have never been taught about fasting, they will do it to heal their bodies naturally.

What are the Spiritual Benefits of fasting? Matthew 17:21 says, *"Some things only come out through fasting and praying."* There are times when we cannot get our breakthrough without putting our flesh under the subjection of the Holy Spirit. Why do we need to place our flesh under subjection? For the Spiritual Purification process.

As a *Bootylicious Queen*, here are a few reasons to fast, but not limited to such:

- ☐ It is vital to use it for our Spiritual Growth.
- ☐ It is vital to use it when we have messed up.
- ☐ It is vital to use it before making any major decisions.
- ☐ It is vital to use it when we encounter negative situations.
- ☐ It is vital to use it when we have been shifted to the core.
- ☐ It is vital to use it when we are sick.
- ☐ It is vital to use it when dealing with difficult people.
- ☐ It is vital to use it when fine-tuning our approaches.
- ☐ It is vital to use it when we are interceding.
- ☐ It is vital to use it when we are clueless.
- ☐ It is vital to use it when we are SPIRITUALLY TESTED.
- ☐ It is vital to use it when suffering from challenges.
- ☐ It is vital to use it when being chastened.
- ☐ It is vital to use it when seeking Spiritual Instructions.
- ☐ It is vital to use it when needing Divine Intervention.
- ☐ It is vital to use it when feeling tempted or lured.
- ☐ It is vital to use it to become better as opposed to bitter.

The Bootylicious Freedom

Fasting is good, but it can become detrimental if we use it to control, manipulate, and deceive others. Here are a few ways fasting will work against us:

- ☐ When we fast to hurt someone. Spiritually, this is a quick way to get hurt or create a generational curse. To unjustly fast to cause harm is very wicked, and one must repent of this sort of wayward behavior.

- ☐ When we fast to force God's hand on a matter without allowing His Divine Will to be done.

- ☐ When we fast out of selfishness. Selfish gain has a way of cursing our hand instead of BLESSING it.

- ☐ When we fast to show off. Using God as a pawning tool will cause us to bring shame to our names quicker than just not fasting at all. Trust me, God knows the intent of the heart; if we think we can fool Him, we are only fooling ourselves instead.

When to Start a Fast?

A fast is designed to teach discipline. Therefore, if we would like our fast to become effective, we must set a marker, which is a designated time to renew our fasting vows through prayer.

As it relates to the wailing process, fasting alone without prayer is basically going without something with no target or destination Spiritually. The fast we are dealing with in this book requires repentance and prayer.

The overall Spiritual Goal is to go without to bring forth or take down. To do so, we must learn the powerful secrets of

The Bootylicious Freedom

fasting. Listed below are a few Spiritual Markers to allow us to realign ourselves with God:

The Sunset Marker: This is a fast from 6 a.m. to 6 a.m. or 6 a.m. to 6 p.m., lasting in 12 or 24-hour increments. This fast can be renewed daily at 6 a.m. or 6 p.m. with an option to vary the fast if needed. Symbolically, this is done for Spiritual Elevation, if we need more of something, such as favor, provision, etc. This viable option is designed to bring more of whatever we so desire **INTO** our lives.

The Noonday Marker: This is a fast from 12 p.m. Noontime to 12 a.m. Midnight or 12 p.m. Noon until 12 pm Noon, the following day, lasting in 12 or 24-hour increments. Symbolically, this fast is done to bring down something. If we need to rid ourselves of something or someone, it is best to choose this fast. This viable option is designed to remove whatever we so desire **OUT** of our lives.

The 7th Hour Marker: These **THREE FASTS** are from 6 a.m. to 12:59 p.m. to bring forth newness, 12:00 p.m. Noon to 6:59 p.m. to take down or remove, or 6 p.m. to 12:59 p.m. to bring forth and remove. This fast only allows you to consume foods going into the 7th hour. What this means is that you would consume a meal at 1 p.m., 7 p.m., or 1:00 a.m. The 6 p.m. to 12:59 a.m. **7th Hour Marker** is the most popular. It is also said to be the easiest, because most people are sleep at around 10-11 p.m.; therefore, they do not feel deprived while getting the same amount of benefits. Plus, they are not going to break their sleep to get up at 1:00 a.m. to eat. However, one must decide what works best and stick to it!

Why the 7th hour and not at 6:00 p.m.? I am basing this off the principle of the 7th Heaven. Is the 7th Heaven Biblical? Of course, Heavenly Places are real, often referred to as the Kingdom of Heaven. Let us take it to scripture anyway: *"And God called the firmaments Heaven. And there was evening and there was morning, the second day."* Genesis 1:8. Spiritually, this is a Realm of the Spirit for Him, *As It Pleases Him*, and being that we are trapped in time, we must RESPECT the Heavenly of Heavens. *"For by Him all things were created that are in heaven and that are on earth, visible and invisible, whether thrones or dominions or principalities or powers. All things were created through Him and for Him."* Colossians 1:16.

We are mere Vessels of Spirituality, regardless of our deed, creed, or breed. Contrary to what most would think, we are not of ourselves. So, if we desire to become divided from something or someone, or bring forth something or someone, in the holiest, purest, and happiest state of mind with extreme JOY, any one of the three Spiritual Markers will work. The ultimate bliss of having an unexplainable inner joy and peace is food for the soul. We do not need to make this complicated; the goal is to get closer to God, period!

Choices of Fasting

Instead of waiting for a once-a-year Day of Fasting, we can create a once-a-week *Day of Fasting*, a *Monthly Fast*, or a *Chamber Fast*. Our soul is considered to be the lifeline. If we can sacrifice 24-25 hours, from sundown to sundown of the following day, to put our flesh under subjection, we would be amazed at the results we would have. As scripture would have it, *"The words of the Lord in the ears of the people in the Lord's house upon the fasting day: and also thou shalt read them in the ears of all Judah that come out of their cities."* Jeremiah 36:6.

Whatever we are going through or going to, our one-day fasting will help us in ways we could not imagine. It will also

The Bootylicious Freedom

bring things to the light regarding what we may have consciously or subconsciously blocked out or suppressed. But more importantly, when we become true to ourselves, we are better able to deal with life and people, and we are better able to take the good with the bad and keep it moving in the Spirit of Excellence.

☐ WEEKLY FAST

This particular fast is where you stop eating one day a week at sundown on Friday at 6 p.m. On Saturday, you can only have juice, broth, smoothies, and water until 6 p.m., and back to normal from Sunday through Thursday. This fast gives your digestive system a break weekly. Why not 7 p.m., according to the 7th Hour Marker Fast? We can choose any of them, but the goal of this fast is more for the long-term, and the 7th Hour is primarily for short-term use to usher in or bring down something.

Above all, we can develop our own schedule, simply take it to God in prayer, *Spirit to Spirit*, seeking what is best for the situation at hand, *As It Pleases Him*. We do not need to overcomplicate this fast; it is between our Heavenly Father and us; therefore, allow the Spirit of the Lord to lead, according to our Predestined Blueprinted Mission.

☐ MONTHLY FAST

The Monthly Fast is the First Fruits fast. This fast is where we sacrifice the first three days of the month to Spiritually Atone the rest of the month, similar to Spiritually Anointing our homes with the Blood of Jesus, but this is for the body. When we give our system a break, we can only have juice, water, smoothies, or vegetable broth. Those with a medical condition must engage in an abridged version according to their doctor's advice.

☐ CHAMBER FAST

The Chamber Fast is the 3, 7, 21, or 40-day absolute, normal, partial, or behavioral fast. However, the length of time is not set in stone. Seek God, *Spirit to Spirit*, regarding the length of time for the fast, *As It Pleases Him*.

The Chamber of Fasting

There are many different chambers of fasting we do not understand; therefore, we give up after only a few hours of trying to fast. In this chapter, each chamber will be broken down accordingly.

What is a chamber? I consider a chamber to be a certain place or room of fasting. If we put our house (the body) on a cold-turkey fast, it may work against us; therefore, if we section the fast off into certain chambers, we can work our way up to the ultimate fast. Remember, each chamber of fasting is still a fast; therefore, God will reward our efforts until we become a pro at this.

Once we have graduated through the chambers, we cannot give God Chamber 1 when we are at Chamber 5. Or, if we are at a Chamber 7 and we want to play in Chamber 1. It does not work like that...once we get through the chambers, it increases our Spirituality to the next level. God will not tolerate us begging Him for His DIVINE BLESSINGS, especially when we are half-stepping in our sacrifices!

When first embarking upon a fast for the first time, one must start slowly. If we have never fasted before, there is a lot of toxic sludge in the body that will make us very sick if we move too fast. To maximize the benefits of fasting, I suggest

The Bootylicious Freedom

starting gradually, with each chamber lasting seven days. Please check with your doctor before beginning any sort of fast.

☐ CHAMBER 1

Removing caffeine first. Yes, this includes soda, coffee, tea, and chocolate. Why? Caffeine keeps our bodies stimulated. If we take out the stimulant in addition to food, we may not survive a fast. Therefore, we must take it very slow....removing a few things at a time to ensure our bodies can adjust to each chamber of the fast. We may experience headaches or dizziness due to the withdrawal of caffeine, but it will subside.

☐ CHAMBER 2

Remove all dairy products, including Chamber 1. We may experience a bad taste in our mouths. All we need to do is brush our teeth and move on.

☐ CHAMBER 3

Remove all forms of meat, including Chambers 1 and 2. It includes all fish, poultry, beef, pork, turkey, and eggs. Yes, I said eggs. Any animal products or anything from an animal must be eliminated in this chamber. However, we may have protein powdered supplements. Once we eliminate meat products, the body will start purifying itself.

☐ CHAMBER 4

Remove all bread, pasta, wheat, cookies, crackers, processed foods, and any inconspicuous gluten, including Chambers 1, 2, and 3.

The Bootylicious Freedom

☐ **CHAMBER 5**
Remove all sugar and starchy products, including Chambers 1, 2, 3, and 4. Sugary products include candy, gum, artificial sweeteners, etc. Starchy products include all types of rice, potatoes, yams, etc. At this point, we are limited to just fruits and non-starchy vegetables.

☐ **CHAMBER 6**
Remove all fruits, including Chambers 1, 2, 3, 4, and 5. Edible fruits must be eliminated at this point. At this stage of the fast, eat only vegetables and drink juice or water.

☐ **CHAMBER 7**
Remove all vegetables, including Chambers 1, 2, 3, 4, 5, and 6. Drink only juice or water.

The *Bootylicious Body* Chamber Fast is second to none, especially for those who are not accustomed to fasting and those who are seeking Divine Refuge and Hope. This Chambered Concept is derived from Isaiah 26:20. *"Come, my people, enter your chambers, and shut your doors behind you; hide yourself, as it were, for a little moment, until the indignation is past."*

Listen to me, and listen well, my *Bootylicious Queen*, there is Spiritual Safety, Comfort, and Protection in becoming Divinely Chambered, *As It Pleases God*. If you allow God to shut the door on people, places, and things that are not conducive to your well-being or Divine Purpose, no one, and I mean no one, can stop the Will of God in your life. Nevertheless, it is your responsibility to ENTER the Divine Chambers of God, *Spirit to Spirit*.

The Bootylicious Freedom

How do we break a fast? When we break our fast, we must regulate ourselves. We must limit the intake of food, taming the monster of gluttony unleashed when we start eating again. Why must we move slowly when breaking a fast? We do not want to overeat or get sick. Plus, the goal is to exercise discipline, so we must adjust our bodies to eating again.

The best way I would suggest is to reverse the chambers, adding food back into our diet in reverse order. For example, if we are in Chamber 7, when we break our fast, we must introduce Chamber 6 back in, then Chamber 5, Chamber 4, Chamber 3, etc. We do not need to introduce all the chambers back in. We have the option to exclude the ones we are comfortable leaving out.

Just so we are clear, regardless of which one we choose when fasting, here are a few things we may encounter at first:

- ☐ We may experience a headache or tiredness.
- ☐ We may experience feeling light-headed or dizzy at times.
- ☐ We may experience aches, cramps, or pains in our bodies.
- ☐ We may experience a body odor change.
- ☐ We may experience constipation.
- ☐ We may go to the bathroom a lot.
- ☐ We may experience bad breath.
- ☐ We may get a little disoriented.
- ☐ We may experience inner or outer chaos.
- ☐ We may experience lucid dreams.
- ☐ We may experience a desire to explore life outside of ourselves.

Nevertheless, we must not give up; these are all the signs of a fast working to purify our bodies of the toxins sitting around hanging out. If we persist, the side effects will go away after three days, but we will have to stay on top of the bad breath

The Bootylicious Freedom

issue and drink lots of water. As a simple reminder, we need water to ensure we do not become dehydrated. Now, here are a few things we need to do when fasting:

- ☐ Limit distractions and noise.
- ☐ Limit Television and Radio.
- ☐ Build a system around your fasting to keep you on track.
- ☐ Follow God's instructional or instinctual nudges.
- ☐ Take notes while praying, and be ready to take notes at any given moment when fasting.
- ☐ Engage in stimulating conversations only.
- ☐ Engage in things you enjoy doing.
- ☐ Do not debate over people, places, and things you cannot change.
- ☐ Keep everything simple and to the point.
- ☐ Create a No-Fight Zone. Focus on peace, love, and happiness.
- ☐ Keep a smile on your face even if you feel as if you have nothing to smile about...smile anyway.

In or out of the *Bootylicious Dietal Plan*, the *Eternal Plan* of God is already established with its own Predestined Blueprint; therefore, we must master creating a win-win situation out of everything.

We are a part of the Divine Plan, so the health of our well-being should not be prolonged. If we need to head into the Spiritual Classroom, do it. If we need to change our perceptions, do it. We are on a Spiritual Mission to set the captives free through Spiritual Empowerment, opening doors that would not have opened otherwise to embrace *The Bootylicious Freedom* of our Forefathers.

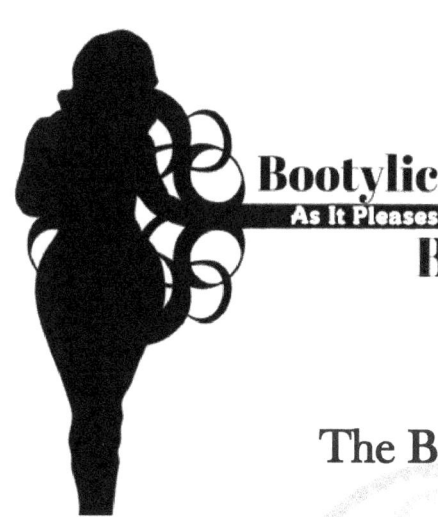

Bootylicious
As It Pleases God
Body

CHAPTER 11

The Bootylicious Meal Plan

Food is designed to fuel us, and anything that God created, He said it was good. Keep in mind that with all of the processed food on the market today, we must go back to the simple fact-finding question that one must ask: *Is it God-Made, or is it man-made?*

My *Bootylicious Queen*, I am indeed a Bush Queen at heart...I believe in using God's natural roots, seeds, fruits, vegetables, nuts, and herbs to nourish, cleanse, and heal the body. If we have excess body fat that is not conducive to our body type or frame, we are eating the wrong foods or not eating the right foods. What does Bush mean? It means using natural herbs or plant-based products. All cultures knowingly or unknowingly use natural herbs.

Some cultures take using herbs out of context without realizing that we use herbs to season our foods, we use herbs for teas, we use herbs in perfumes, we use herbs in medicine, we use herbs in body care products, we use herbs in cleaning products; basically, we use herbs in everything. Most often,

The Bootylicious Meal Plan

the small amount of herbs that we get in seasoning our foods and other various ways may not be enough to heal, cleanse, and nourish the body. Therefore, we must understand how to make herbal remedies work on our behalf without falling into the trap of misunderstanding what God has given us to heal ourselves.

Herbal products are now in great demand! We have finally recognized that herbs are healing, cleansing, and renewing people in a natural way. As we know, results are not immediate; they are subtle but effective and long-lasting. Nevertheless, as God would have it, there are a lot of herbal products on the market now, but you must be ever so cognizant of the side effects. Too much of anything is not good!

Natural, organic food is healthier and better for your digestive system. Regardless of whether we believe in the bush or not, *The Bootylicious Body* is very symbolic due to the fact that Man was created in the Bible on the 6th day. Most do not recognize the number 6 as being symbolic because they have some sort of taboo related to it. However, *The Bootylicious Body* is going to reveal how symbolic the number is and how it can help us take charge of our lives without having a man-made negative stigma associated.

The next reason for six being symbolic for us is that God took 6 days to create everything and took the 7th day to rest. In my opinion, this lets us know how important it is to rest our bodies at least one day out of the week.

For *The Bootylicious Body*, we follow the same principle. We use the structured plan for 6 days, and on the 7th day, we must rest our bodies. Thus, creating a free day to eat whatever we so desire or fast. Furthermore, as a part of our structure, timing is everything. We have an eating schedule that will allow us to only consume certain types of food based on the widely used time clock.

The Bootylicious Meal Plan

To make it very simple, if we look at the clock closely, in the morning, the hour shorthand is going up, and in the afternoon, the hour shorthand is going down in 6-hour increments.

In the morning, we want to raise our level of Spirituality symbolically in that 6-hour increment from **6:00 a.m. in the Morning – 12:00 p.m. NOON**. Unbeknown to most, this is when our bodies will absorb the most amount of nutrients, so this is when we want to take our vitamins and supplements.

Then in the evening, from **6:00 p.m. – 12:00 a.m. Midnight**, we can only partake of foods that will increase our level of consciousness when the short arrow on the clock is rising. **NO HEAVY FOODS.** According to our Divine Design, this is when our bodies begin to relax by default.

Now, from **12:00 p.m. NOON – 6:00 p.m. in the Evening**, we will find that the shorthand arrow goes downward, and our ultimate goal is to lose weight. Symbolically, we can only eat regular foods during this time to ensure that we are mentally lining up our bodies to lose weight. Or better yet, allowing the pounds to fall off.

From **12:00 a.m. Midnight – 6:00 a.m. in the Morning** is mandatory rest—MEANING NO FOOD.

The Clock Short Rising

The Clock Short Hand Falling

Once you understand the power of the clock or the power of timing from a *SYMBOLIC* standpoint, you are ready to begin

The Bootylicious Meal Plan

The Bootylicious Body. If you have Dietary Supplements, take them 30 minutes prior to your meal. You can also start your day with *The Bootylicious Body* Miracle Blend, which is available online at: www.BootyliciousBody.com.

A *SERVING* is the size of the palm of your hand unless otherwise stated. Your self-contained measuring cup forces you to begin to eyeball your food portions instinctively to ensure your success publicly or privately.

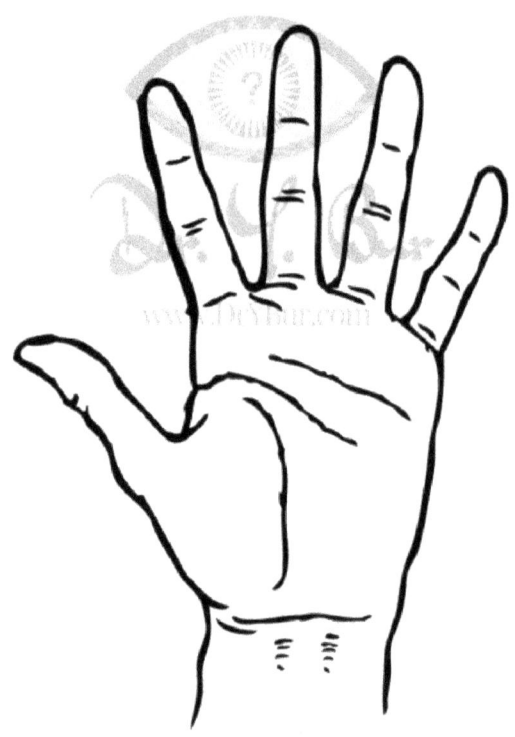

The Bootylicious Meal Plan

For Breakfast

The Bootylicious Body keeps our meal plan very simple. Choose 1 Fruit and 1 Food Item from *the Bootylicious Body* **Breakfast List**. Or, choose 1 Fruit and 1 serving of *The Bootylicious Body* Miracle Blend mixed into a smoothie for breakfast. Then, for your morning snack, choose 1 Fruit and 1 Dairy Item from *the Bootylicious Body* Food List. (*Items are Diabetic Approved)

"The Bootylicious Body" Breakfast List
6:00 a.m. – 12:00 p.m.

Choose **TWO** Fruit Items:

- Apple*
- Grapefruit*
- Lime*
- Cranberries*
- Lemon*
- Mango
- Orange*
- Papaya*
- Peaches
- Pineapples*
- Coconut*
- Pomegranate
- Soursop*
- Avocado*

- Dragon or Star Fruit
- Passion Fruit
- Blackberries
- Acai Berries
- Pears*

Choose **One Starch or Protein** Item:

- Oatmeal or Quinoa*
- Cream of Wheat
- Grits
- *The Bootylicious Body* Miracle Blend Smoothie *
- Protein Shake*.

The Bootylicious Meal Plan

"The Bootylicious Body"
Snack List
6:00 a.m. – 12:00 p.m.

Choose **ONE** Fruit Item:

- ☐ Apple*
- ☐ Grapefruit*
- ☐ Lime*
- ☐ Cranberries*
- ☐ Lemon*
- ☐ Mango
- ☐ Orange*
- ☐ Papaya*
- ☐ Peaches
- ☐ Pineapples*
- ☐ Coconut*
- ☐ Pomegranate
- ☐ Soursop*
- ☐ Avocado*
- ☐ Dragon Fruit
- ☐ Passion Fruit
- ☐ Blackberries
- ☐ Starfruit
- ☐ Acai Berries
- ☐ Pears*
- ☐ Cherries
- ☐ Cantaloupe
- ☐ Honeydew Melon
- ☐ Kiwi
- ☐ Watermelon
- ☐ Grapes

Choose **ONE** Dairy Item:

- ☐ Skim Milk
- ☐ Soy Milk
- ☐ Almond Milk*
- ☐ Cottage Cheese*
- ☐ Cheese*
- ☐ Yogurt*

If you get hungry before lunch or dinner, simply have Jell-O or eat an extra apple.

- ☐ Extra Apple
- ☐ Jell-O

The Bootylicious Meal Plan

For Lunch and Dinner

All portions must fit in your saucer plate; therefore, you must leave room for your veggies and grains that can only be consumed between the hours of **12:00 p.m. Noon, and 6 p.m., in the Evening.**

The Bootylicious Body suggested time for eating is 1 meal at **12:00 p.m., Noonday,** and 1 meal at **5:00 p.m., in the Evening**. However, the choice is yours regarding what time you will eat between the hours of **12:00 p.m. and 6 p.m.** For each meal, you are able to have:

- *1 PROTEIN*
- *1 STARCH*
- *2 OR 3 VEGETABLES*
- *1 FAT*

During these 2 structured meals, '*The Bootylicious Body*' does not allow the consumption of fruits or desserts while having your meal. However, you are able to have certain fruits as a snack in between your meals during the hours of **12:00 p.m. Noonday and 6 p.m., in the Evening.**

This plan is NOT designed to deprive you; it is designed to bring BALANCE to your body while provoking your body to burn the unwanted fat that is needed to get your body to its natural set point.

For Diabetics: Managing diabetes effectively requires a comprehensive approach to nutrition, with careful consideration of how food choices impact blood sugar levels. As a *Bootylicious Queen*, one effective strategy for diabetics is the order in which they consume their food. Specifically, eating

The Bootylicious Meal Plan

vegetables first, followed by healthy fats, and then protein, before indulging in starches, can help mitigate blood sugar spikes. Still, with your fat portion, you have the option to choose how you will use it when preparing your protein, starch, or veggies.

"The Bootylicious Body" Regular Food Choices
12:00 p.m. – 6:00 p.m.

Choose **ONE** Serving of Protein for Lunch and Dinner:

- ☐ Beans
- ☐ Chicken
- ☐ Seafood
- ☐ Eggs
- ☐ Fish
- ☐ Turkey
- ☐ Tofu
- ☐ Nuts
- ☐ Peanut Butter

Choose **ONE** Serving of Starch (Grain) for Lunch or Dinner:

- ☐ Corn
- ☐ White Potatoes
- ☐ Yams
- ☐ Oatmeal
- ☐ Grits
- ☐ Cream of Wheat
- ☐ Sweet Potatoes
- ☐ Pasta
- ☐ Bread
- ☐ Cereal
- ☐ Rice

The Bootylicious Meal Plan

Choose **TWO** or **THREE** Servings of Vegetables for Lunch or Dinner. These vegetables are low in calories and high in vitamins, minerals, and fiber.

- ☐ Asparagus
- ☐ Bean sprouts
- ☐ Broccoli
- ☐ Cabbage
- ☐ Brussel Sprouts
- ☐ Greens (Any Type)
- ☐ Carrots
- ☐ Cauliflower
- ☐ Celery
- ☐ Cucumbers
- ☐ Eggplant
- ☐ Okra
- ☐ Onions
- ☐ Kale
- ☐ Lettuce (various types)
- ☐ Spinach
- ☐ Green Peppers
- ☐ Radishes
- ☐ Rhubarb
- ☐ Squash
- ☐ String Beans
- ☐ Tomato
- ☐ Turnips
- ☐ Zucchini
- ☐ Hot Peppers
- ☐ Garlic
- ☐ Beets
- ☐ Mushrooms
- ☐ Ginger
- ☐ Collard Greens
- ☐ Peas
- ☐ Bok Choy

Choose **ONE** Fat for Lunch and Dinner: *1 Tablespoon Allowed Per Meal*

- ☐ Light Butter
- ☐ Light Mayonnaise
- ☐ Olive Oil
- ☐ Coconut Oil
- ☐ Nut Oil
- ☐ Chia Seeds
- ☐ Flax Seeds

The Bootylicious Meal Plan

"The Bootylicious Body"
Snack List

12:00 p.m. – 6:00 p.m. for Lunch or Dinner

Choose **ONE** Item:

- Apple*
- Grapefruit*
- Lime*
- Cranberries*
- Lemon*
- Mango
- Orange*
- Papaya*
- Peaches
- Pineapples*
- Coconut*
- Pomegranate
- Soursop*
- Avocado*
- Dragon Fruit
- Passion Fruit
- Blackberries
- Starfruit
- Acai Berries
- Pears*
- Cherries
- Cantaloupe
- Honeydew Melon
- Kiwi
- Watermelon
- Grapes

Choose **ONE** Dairy Item:

- Skim Milk
- Soy Milk
- Almond Milk*
- Cottage Cheese*
- Cheese*
- Yogurt*

After 6:00 p.m., in the evening, you are allowed 1 fruit, plenty of water, and herbal tea for the rest of the evening until Midnight. If you get hungry during the night, grab some Jell-O to avoid any self-sabotage. However, after Midnight, you can have absolutely nothing but water until 6:00 a.m.

The Bootylicious Meal Plan

"The Bootylicious Body"
After Hours List
6:00 p.m. – 12:00 a.m.

Choose **ONE** Item:

- Apple*
- Grapefruit*
- Lime*
- Cranberries*
- Lemon*
- Mango
- Orange*
- Papaya*
- Peaches
- Pineapples
- Coconut*
- Pomegranate
- Soursop*
- Jell-O
- Vegetable Smoothie
- All Fruit Smoothie
- Warm Herbal Tea

"The Bootylicious Body"
FREE Items List
6:00 a.m. – 12:00 a.m.

- All Herbs (Cilantro, Parsley, Basil, Oregano, Thyme, Rosemary, Dill, Mint, Chives, Tarragon, Bay Leaves, Lemongrass, etc.) They can be used fresh, dried, or as extracts in cooking and beverages.
- Salt-Free Seasonings.
- The *Bootylicious Body* Salt-Free Seasonings.
- Cinnamon.
- Vanilla extract.

The Bootylicious Meal Plan

Our *Bootylicious Body* Salt-Free Seasonings are designed to keep your sodium intake at an all-time low. One area where many people struggle is managing sodium intake, which can be linked to several health issues, including hypertension 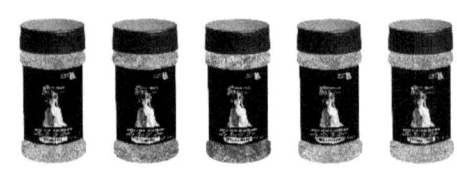 and heart disease. Our *Bootylicious Body* Salt-Free Seasonings are designed to ensure you can savor your bold and delicious flavors without the need for added salt.

Our *Bootylicious Body* Salt-Free Seasonings are meticulously crafted with a blend of herbs, spices, and natural ingredients that elevate the taste of your meals, making every bite a delight. Our diverse range of salt-free seasonings can be used in a variety of dishes, from roasted vegetables to baked meats and even salad dressings. They allow you to experiment with flavors and cuisines without the worry of adding too much sodium.

Using our *Bootylicious Body* Salt-Free Seasonings means you can cook with confidence, knowing that you are making healthy choices for yourself and your loved ones. Whether you are preparing a family dinner or a quick lunch, our seasonings provide the perfect finishing touch to your meals. They are available at www.BootyliciousBody.com.

Here are a few quick recipe ideas to inspire you to incorporate our salt-free seasonings into your cooking:

- ☐ Zesty Roasted Vegetables: Toss your favorite vegetables with olive oil and a generous sprinkle of The *Bootylicious Body* Salt-Free Seasoning of your choice. Roast in the oven until tender and enjoy a delicious, guilt-free side dish.

The Bootylicious Meal Plan

- ☐ Flavorful Grilled Chicken: Marinate chicken breasts in a mix of The *Bootylicious Body* Salt-Free Seasoning of your choice, lemon juice, and olive oil before grilling, baking, or sautéing. Serve with a side of steamed vegetables for a nutritious meal.

- ☐ Savory Quinoa Salad: Cook quinoa and let it cool. Mix with diced cucumbers, tomatoes, and a drizzle of olive oil. Add The *Bootylicious Body* Salt-Free Seasoning of your choice for an explosion of flavor that is low in sodium.

- ☐ Herbed Omelet: Whip up an egg omelet and fill it with your choice of veggies. Sprinkle with The *Bootylicious Body* Salt-Free Seasoning of your choice before folding for a perfectly seasoned breakfast.

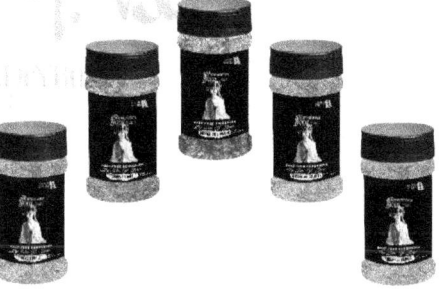

On behalf of Dr. Y. Bur, The WHY Doctor, say goodbye to the bland, salt-heavy meals and embrace a new, delicious way to season your life; one sprinkle at a time!

The bottom line is that this weight management plan works, and if you dedicate yourself to this plan, your body will plateau at its set point with results that you will be pleased with, Guaranteed! Once you become accustomed to eating in such a manner, you will soon find that there is more to life than just existing here on Earth.

Remember to take your time when eating, and enjoy your food by chewing slowly to savor and digest it properly. When you chew your food more thoroughly, you break it down into smaller pieces, which makes it easier for your stomach to digest. Saliva, which is produced as you chew, contains enzymes that begin the digestion process. Simply put, this means that the more you chew, the more effectively your body can absorb nutrients with the active participation of your second brain (Your Digestive System).

Additionally, eating slowly allows your body time to signal fullness to your brain. According to our DNA, it typically takes about 20 minutes for the brain to register that you are full. By slowing down, you give your body the chance to communicate this feeling before you overeat. As a *Bootylicious Queen*, this can help regulate your calorie intake and prevent unnecessary weight gain.

With *The Bootylicious Body* Dietal System, the goal is to transform eating into a mindful experience of enjoyment. Why do we need to turn eating into an experience, especially when eating is a necessity? It reduces our stress levels. If we are in a hurry to eat or are afraid to eat, it increases our stress hormones, such as cortisol, somewhat thwarting the digestion process. For some, this may cause us to pack on the pounds or experience a wide range of digestive issues, including indigestion, bloating, and decreased nutrient absorption.

Conversely, eating in a state of stress can lead to poor food choices. And a fast-paced, on-the-go lifestyle may also lead to habitual overeating and stress-related weight gain if we are not careful. Does this really matter? Absolutely, primarily when we get older and more sedentary, where heart disease and diabetes become more prevalent and problematic.

More importantly, understanding the relationship between how we eat, our stress levels, and the effects of our genetic predispositions can help us make better choices for a healthier lifestyle.

The Bootylicious Meal Plan

With *The Bootylicious Meal Plan*, here is what is desired from a *Bootylicious Queen*, but not limited to such:

- ☐ Set the Scene: Create a calm and pleasant eating environment by reducing distractions. Turn off the TV, put away your phone, and focus on your meal.

- ☐ Put Down the Utensils: Between bites, place your fork or spoon down on the table. This practice encourages you to pause and take a moment to enjoy the flavors before continuing.

- ☐ Take Small Bites: Smaller bites are easier to chew and can help you pace your eating naturally. They also allow you to experience the true essence of your food.

- ☐ Engage Your Senses: Pay attention to the colors, aromas, and textures of your food. This active engagement can enhance your appreciation and enjoyment of the meal.

- ☐ Practice Gratitude: Before eating, take a moment to express gratitude or pray over the food on your plate. This simple practice can set a positive tone for the meal. Remember, every morsel of food is a BLESSING.

So the next time you sit down for a meal, remember to slow down, chew thoughtfully, enjoy each delicious bite, and give thanks. In the Eye of God, this goes a long way, especially when regulating your hormones, *As It Pleases God*.

Now that we have delved into the details of *The Bootylicious Meal Plan*, it is time to turn our attention to another exciting aspect of healthy eating: the *Smoothie Sensation*. With an infinite combination of fruits, vegetables, proteins, and healthy fats, smoothies can serve as a meal replacement, a quick snack, or even a post-workout refuel.

Smoothie Sensation

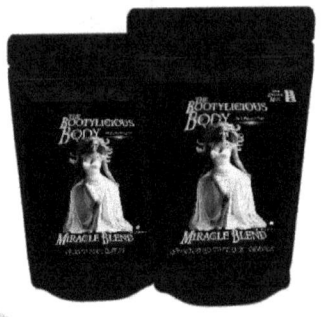

The *Smoothie Sensation* is more than just a trend; it is a lifestyle choice that allows you to pack essential nutrients into a delicious drink.

Smoothies offer a versatile and nutritious alternative meal option that can cater to various tastes and dietary needs. It has been around since the beginning of time, and it is not going anywhere any time soon. It is designed to help stave off hunger and prevent your digestive system from having to work too much. It is good to give your system a break, and it is also a good way to get your fruits and veggies in.

The Bootylicious Body does not advocate processed meal replacement drinks or bar supplements. We want you to learn how to make your own and how to choose natural, unprocessed foods. This is not about taking the easy way out! It is about learning what foods to eat and what foods not to eat. Although some weight loss bars and drink supplements work for some, I want you to learn what works for your body and what does not!

When dieting, smoothies can assist in the cravings for sweets as well, so that you can achieve your weight loss goals. It will also help you when you get hungry in between meals, therefore helping you to stick to your diet plan a little better than going without them. When incorporating smoothies into your health and wellness plan, you will notice that you

The Bootylicious Meal Plan

will have fewer viruses and sicknesses in your body while losing weight at the same time.

Our bodies require certain nutrients, and if we do not have the appropriate nutrients in our bodies, we can become malnourished without even realizing that we are. When we appear healthy, but severely malnourished, it can go undetected for years until our organs begin to fail or we become diabetic or suffer from hypertension. When our bodies have to overwork to produce certain nutrients or insulin to keep us alive, it becomes overworked, causing hypertensiveness in those who are not eating properly, those who are eating the wrong foods for their body, or those who are not eating enough food for the size of their body. When we become hypertensive or diabetic, it will become harder to lose weight simply because our bodies have become conditioned to keep us alive, and it will resist certain foods. Therefore, it is best that if you are diabetic or hypertensive, you check with your doctor before implementing smoothies into your diet.

Smoothies that are typically higher in sugar, especially those made with certain fruits, sweeteners, or added juices, can cause spikes in glucose levels. Instead, choosing low-glycemic fruits such as berries, along with incorporating sources of protein (like Greek yogurt or nuts) and healthy fats (like avocado), can help stabilize blood sugar responses. As *Bootylicious Queens*, here are a few benefits of the *Smoothie Sensation*, but not limited to such:

- ☐ They are Nutrient-Dense: Smoothies can be loaded with vitamins, minerals, and antioxidants, providing you with a powerful health boost. Incorporating leafy greens, berries, and nut-based yogurt can significantly increase your intake of essential nutrients.

The Bootylicious Meal Plan

- ☐ They are Customizable: No two smoothies have to be the same! You can tailor your smoothie according to your dietary preferences and goals. Whether you are vegan, gluten-free, or looking for a protein-packed option, the possibilities are endless.

- ☐ They Aid in Convenience: In today's fast-paced world, smoothies offer a time-efficient way to get a wholesome meal. Preparing your ingredients the night before makes it easy to whip up a nutritious blend in just a few minutes.

- ☐ They Aid in Digestion: Smoothies made from fiber-rich fruits and vegetables can help promote healthy digestion. Adding ingredients like chia seeds or flaxseeds can further enhance digestive health while providing a good dose of omega-3 fatty acids.

- ☐ They Aid in Hydration: Many smoothies incorporate liquid bases like coconut water, almond milk, or even plain water, helping you stay hydrated while enjoying a meal.

Now, the question is, 'Can diet reverse diabetes and hypertension?' The answer is Yes. However, you must tread carefully, and you cannot go off your medication with the 'Cold Turkey' philosophy. When you begin to eat the right foods for your body and drink healthy smoothies, it will change your life for the better.

My *Bootylicious Queen*, you must understand that your body is different from the next person, and there is no need to compare yourself to someone else. Your body will tell you

The Bootylicious Meal Plan

what it likes and what it does not—you simply need to pay attention and listen to your body. If a particular food spikes your sugar or blood pressure, that is an automatic sign that it is not conducive to your body type. Although your body can adapt to any food in the midst of famine, it will stress your body, causing undue pressure or sickness. Plus, we are not in the midst of a famine; therefore, if our body says no, then it should be a NO!

My *Bootylicious Queen*, it is best to replace evening meals or a meal on the run with smoothies; nevertheless, you must find what works for you. Some people sleep better with a fuller tummy, and some cannot sleep well on an emptier tummy. Moreover, find your smoothie niche, make it work for you, and stick to it. Make sure you add *The Bootylicious Body* Miracle Blend to your smoothie as well. It is available online at: www.BootyliciousBody.com.

To master the art of smoothie-making and to ensure you are getting a well-rounded meal in a glass, here are some tips:

- ☐ Start with a Base: Choose a liquid such as water, coconut water, fruit-flavored tea, fruit juice, or milk (dairy or non-dairy, including soy, oat, cashew, or almond milk) as your smoothie base. One of these bases will help achieve the right consistency that works for you and your taste buds.

- ☐ Add Fruits and Vegetables: Fresh or frozen fruits like bananas, berries, and mangoes add natural sweetness, while greens such as spinach or kale provide essential nutrients without overpowering the taste.

- ☐ Include Protein: To make your smoothie more filling, consider adding protein sources like Greek yogurt,

The Bootylicious Meal Plan

protein powder, nut butter, or *The Bootylicious Body Miracle Blend*.

☐ Incorporate Healthy Fats: A tablespoon of flaxseeds, chia seeds, avocado oil, or coconut oil can provide healthy fats, helping you stay satisfied longer.

☐ Experiment with Flavors: Do not hesitate to get creative! Adding spices like cinnamon, ginger, or even a dash of vanilla extract can elevate the flavor profile of your smoothie.

Above all, in all of your *Bootyliciousness*, find a way to *Jazz It Up*, and your taste buds will thank you!

Jazz It Up

This book, *The Bootylicious Body*, is not a diet of punishment; it is a diet of renewal. It is designed to help you understand how you were created. Having the perfect body is a matter of perception based on our mindset, culture, or tradition. As long as you believe that you are good enough for you...then that is all that matters. What people think is their problem, and what you think about you is yours, right? Absolutely. The goal is health and longevity.

Do not ever get into the mindset that food is bad for you! Simply set in your mind that processed food is unwise for the body. When you do not know what is in your food, it becomes a problem. It is imperative that you know what you are eating. If you are clueless about what you are eating, then it becomes harder to predict the results.

The problem is that we eat the wrong foods and we gain weight, which causes us to fear all food. The fear of the great

The Bootylicious Meal Plan

unknown has become an epidemic. We do not know what we are eating, and our emotional fear is eating us from the inside out.

How can eating become a witch-hunt for the human race? We are designed to eat good, natural, and bountiful food, and now everything is fast, fast, fast, and nutrient-free! No one wants to cook, and everyone wants to lose weight.

Our bodies are starving, and we do not even realize it. Our bodies are not getting bigger because of real, natural food. It is getting bigger due to eating processed or synthetic food, the lack of nutrients, the lack of water, and the lack of exercise. When we overeat, our bodies should be pooping it out. If we are not, then where is the food going? Is it just sitting there?

What happens to meat when it is left sitting outside in 100-degree temperatures? Yet, no one is educating us on this. If our digestive tract is blocked with too much garbage, then the food sits in our bodies, getting stored as fat and toxic sludge. Unfortunately, this happens because the body is overworking itself to keep up with the demands of trying to get the nutrients out of the next meal. Now, with this same cycle continuing for years, how big or sick will we become with garbage in our digestive tract? My point exactly...my goal is to get you to think!

Foods that are the closest to their natural state are good for you. If you jazz it up with a few herbs and spices, it makes food a little exciting. The key to *The Bootylicious Body* is proper portions and moderation. You do not have to sacrifice flavor in order to diet; you simply need to avoid foods that are processed. We also need to learn how to substitute certain ingredients for healthier ones, such as how butter can be replaced with coconut oil. Dipping sauces and dressings can be made from the juice of certain vegetables. The goal is to

The Bootylicious Meal Plan

bring you back to a healthier tradition, as opposed to the new-age tradition of processing everything.

Cucumbers, peppers, broccoli, celery, and carrot sticks are all healthy snacks that are easily accessible. So, do not be fooled by the prepackaged processed snack packs...if it is not fruits, nuts, or veggies in their natural or dried state, then it may not be a wise choice of snacks. Therefore, it behooves you to be in the know when it comes down to what is going into your body and the reasons why.

In my opinion, when we are in the know about things, life becomes easier for us, even if we cannot have our way. The goal is to remain positive, focused, and ready, while everything else works itself out for the Greater Good as we become *Naturally Bootylicious*.

Dr. Y. Bur

www.DrYBur.com

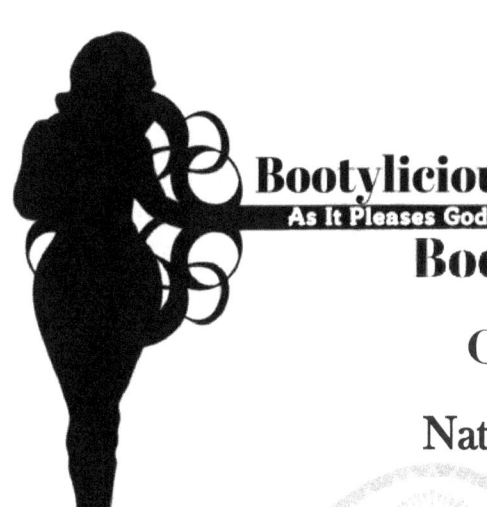

CHAPTER 12
Naturally Bootylicious

Once you begin to eat more *Natural* foods, you will have an instant improvement in your self-confidence, resulting in weight loss. Here is how it works: Once you release the stress, your body will naturally begin to lose weight due to the balancing of your hormones. When your hormones are unbalanced, it is normal to gain or lose weight, depending on your genetic makeup. For a *Bootylicious Queen*, unbalanced hormones mean weight gain!

The relationship between patients and healthcare professionals is vital; however, the dynamic can sometimes lead to feelings of inadequacy, particularly when it involves weight and body image. I have had a healthcare professional document in my records with an opening statement saying: 'This is an obese African American woman.' It was not a diagnosis; it was a blatant statement as if I would not read the notes. But of course, I read everything! Every interaction, from the initial consultation to follow-up appointments, shapes a patient's understanding of their condition and overall experience. Unfortunately, there are instances where the clarity of communication is overshadowed by assumptions, biases, or oversights.

I could have gotten offended with a point of correction, saying, 'I am an obese Afro-Cherokee Bootylicious Black Woman.' But of course, he had no clue who he was insulting, so I did not take it personally—and there was no need to get petty. Besides, my Mom and I got a good laugh out of it, and now here we are...this story made it into *The Bootylicious Body: As It Pleases God*®.

I am not saying to avoid or not listen to your healthcare professional. I am saying do not allow them to crush your self-confidence because they think that you are too fat or overweight due to your ethnicity, especially if their eating habits may be worse than yours. The cycle of shame and guilt can cause you to second-guess your diet, feel unworthy of attention, or even avoid medical visits altogether. Remember, as a *Bootylicious Queen*, your value is not determined by a number on a scale or someone else's perception of your body or cultural background. Good health is the goal while letting no one or nothing prevent you from celebrating your small victories.

How would a person deal with this issue in a nice way? Simply, ask them about their eating habits and what foods help them to maintain their weight. More than likely, they will stumble over their words or redirect the question. If so, then you automatically know that they have bad eating habits as well, and they are passing judgment on you, primarily when they may be genetically thinner according to their DNA structure.

As *Bootylicious Queens*, when being *Naturally Bootylicious*, body shaming will come with the territory, regardless of our shapes, sizes, and backgrounds. So, in the Eye of God, it is wise to build our character positively, while using the Fruits of the Spirit consistently to offset the mocking, belittling, judging, criticizing, or hurtful comments. If not, the emotional stress will cause self-esteem issues or long-term mental issues. All of which leads to packing on the pounds or stress eating, along with a myriad of negative emotional responses that surround feelings of being ashamed, embarrassed, depressed, isolated, or anxious.

Why would negative emotions engulf us as Believers who are Naturally Bootylicious? The reason is not set in stone because we are all different, with varying issues and experiences. Nonetheless, the constant pressure to conform to societal ideals can become overwhelming, triggering our unresolved issues and traumas from within. If not resolved, *As It Pleases God*, the undue pressures may result in some type of underlying eating disorder or becoming a body shamer ourselves. Then again, we may constantly and secretly feel as if we are not good enough, or make other people feel as such through projecting and deflecting. Can this really happen to us? It is happening in real time, especially in our social circles, fashion standards, social media, cultural standards, and with familial expectations.

This body-shaming phenomenon underscores a need for body positivity, even if we are thinner or thicker than the norm. My *Bootylicious Queen*, embracing body diversity and fostering self-love, are crucial steps toward healing, *As It Pleases God*. As we redefine what it means to be beautiful and *Naturally Bootylicious*, our bodies tell a story that no one can take from us.

Self-love is indeed the Divine Cornerstone of our healing, as compassion, kindness, and understanding become our portion, leaving self-doubt and biases where they belong— under our feet. As we move forward in the Spirit of Excellence, we take our talents, creativity, strengths, uniqueness, and Birthrights with us to fulfill our reason for being, even if it jiggles a little or a lot!

From one *Bootylicious Queen* to another, you are beautiful in the skin you are in; you may need to make better choices in selecting the right foods for your body type, but you are the best version of yourself, and God did not make a mistake when making you *Bootylicious* and Fabulous.

The Bootylicious Connection

My Bootylicious *Queen*, being able to handle the stresses of life is predicated on us being properly equipped with knowledge, wisdom, and understanding. Therefore, we must take time out to relax, exercise, and balance ourselves appropriately. When it is all said and done, we need peace of mind in order to become successful at losing weight and keeping it off. Plus, it also helps to keep our emotional triggers in check. As a matter of fact, if we add a little exercise into our daily routine, we will find that it will raise our self-esteem, motivation, and willpower, preventing us from becoming easily crushed by negativity and silent abuse.

In creating a pleasing lifestyle as a *Bootylicious Queen* and *As It Pleases God* demands a heart and mind posture of authenticity. It does not matter how much you have or do not have; the authentic you will win every single time. Still, you must know and understand this factor beyond a shadow of a doubt. If there is any doubt lingering within the psyche, you can create a disservice to the Mind, Body, Soul, and Spirit. So, it behooves you to stick to being yourself, *As It Pleases God*.

In *The Bootylicious Connection*, you are God's PRIZE, and under no circumstance should you dim the Light of God inside of you. From this point forward, I need you to move forward in the Spirit of Excellence, allowing nothing or no one to zap the Greatness lying within you. Yes, you! I do not care what it looks like...I am telling you how it is in the Eye of God.

You have what it takes to achieve or accomplish anything you so desire; you need only to BELIEVE without stealing the shine of another. Remember, you are BLESSED with Light to Divinely Illuminate others. The more you give it, the brighter you will become Mentally, Physically, Emotionally, Spiritually, and Financially.

With the *Bootylicious Body* granted to you from the Heavenly of Heavens, you are designed to carry the Weight of Greatness because you are the stronger VESSEL full of Virtue, Creativity, and Wisdom. Without further ado, now is the time to bring forth that which is already shut up in your loins for a time such as this.

The powerful force inside each of us represents the Divine Essence of God, and the moment we forget who we are, we can indeed hinder our virtues of resilience, compassion, and creativity. Yes, you may have to work harder, but you can also work smarter with God in the midst of whatever with whomever.

Listen, you are *Naturally Bootylicious* for a reason, not to merely celebrate physical beauty, but to rejoice in the internal beauty with the Chosen People in the Body of Christ. Thus, it is also your responsibility to remove your deceitful grave clothes of mediocrity. Furthermore, for this Divine Wisdom, for your sake, I did not go through all of the trials, tribulations, setbacks, and abuses for nothing. Nor should you allow it to go in vain; someone had to get it, and I made the sacrifice to do so to feed God's sheep. If you are a sheep of the Kingdom, get yourself up and get ready to stand tall in your *Bootyliciousness*, taking all of the Divine Wisdom gained from your life experiences, knowledge, and reflections to help another *Bootylicious Queen*, activating the Law of Reciprocity.

Naturally Bootylicious

The unstoppable POWER is now at your fingertips with the Holy Trinity, Quaternity, and Quinternity working in your favor—oops, that is Divine Favor, to be exact. Why? Science cannot trace your Divine Greatness when approached with such precision. Plus, you will always stay ahead of the game because the Secrets of the Mind are designed to PROTECT you...so, keep people out of your head, use the Fruits of the Spirit, and take your rightful place as the *Bootylicious Queen* that you are. From me to you, my *Bootylicious Queen*, I believe in you...Grow Great! You got this!

Dr. Y. Bur

The Bootylicious Body Diary

Breakfast:

Snack:

Lunch:

Dinner:

Snack:

The Bootylicious Baby Diary

Breakfast:

Snack:

Lunch:

Dinner:

Snack:

The Bootylicious Body Diary

Breakfast:

Snack:

Lunch:

Dinner:

Snack:

The Bootylicious Body Diary

Breakfast:

Snack:

Lunch:

Dinner:

Snack:

The Bootylicious Body Diary

Breakfast:

Snack:

Lunch:

Dinner:

Snack:

The Bootylicious Body Diary

Breakfast:

Snack:

Lunch:

Dinner:

Snack:

The Bootylicious Body Diary

Breakfast:

Snack:

Lunch:

Dinner:

Snack:

The Bootylicious Body Diary

Breakfast:

Snack:

Lunch:

Dinner:

Snack:

The Bootylicious Body Diary

Breakfast:

Snack:

Lunch:

Dinner:

Snack:

The Bootylicious Body Diary

Breakfast:

Snack:

Lunch:

Dinner:

Snack:

The Bootylicious Body Diary

Breakfast:

Snack:

Lunch:

Dinner:

Snack:

The Bootylicious Body Diary

Breakfast:

Snack:

Lunch:

Dinner:

Snack:

The Bootylicious Body Diary

Breakfast:

Snack:

Lunch:

Dinner:

Snack:

The Bootylicious Body Diary

Breakfast:

Snack:

Lunch:

Dinner:

Snack:

The Bootylicious Body Diary

Breakfast:

Snack:

Lunch:

Dinner:

Snack:

The Bootylicious Body Diary

Breakfast:

Snack:

Lunch:

Dinner:

Snack:

The Bootylicious Body Diary

Breakfast:

Snack:

Lunch:

Dinner:

Snack:

The Bootylicious Body Diary

Breakfast:

Snack:

Lunch:

Dinner:

Snack:

The Bootylicious Body Diary

Breakfast:

Snack:

Lunch:

Dinner:

Snack:

The Bootylicious Body Diary

Breakfast:

Snack:

Lunch:

Dinner:

Snack:

www.ingramcontent.com/pod-product-compliance
Lightning Source LLC
Chambersburg PA
CBHW071711160426
43195CB00012B/1645